What do you know about Endorphins?

Did you know —

✓ That Endorphins are your own biochemical regulators of pain-relief, joy, and well-being?

✓ That you can stimulate your own Endorphins— even through your thoughts and feelings?

✓ That you can block your Endorphin flow of happiness because of preconditioned thoughts, feelings, and beliefs?

✓ That, because of Endorphins' opiate-like action, you can, over time, build up a numbing tolerance to your own euphoric Endorphin experience?

✓ Because of this potential for adaptation, life can become routine and boring. But we can prevent this process from occurring.

✓ No longer must we be the victims of outer circumstances or the followers of another's dogma. Each of us has power and resources *from within* — to experience life in its fullest dimension—to make each day better than the last—each moment of time more lovely.

✓ Not just another panacea, Endorphin information and its practiced application empowers you with the tools you need to influence your health and create your own happiness.

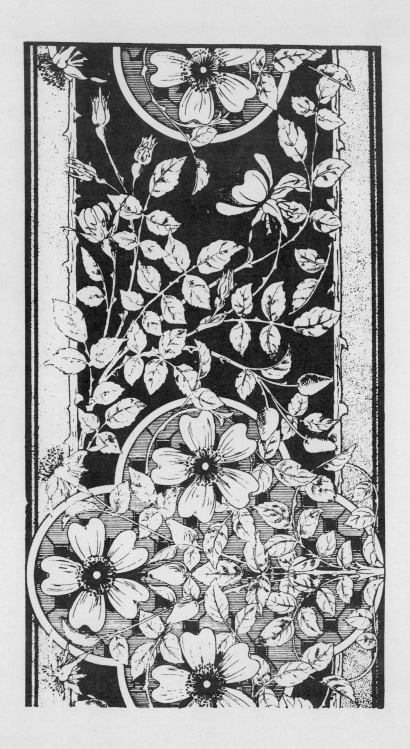

THE PLEASURE CONNECTION

How Endorphins Affect Our Health and Happiness

Deva Beck, R.N. & James Beck, R.N.

FOREWORD BY
Dr. C. Norman Shealy, M.D., Ph.D.

SYNTHESIS PRESS

Library of Congress Cataloging in Publication Data
Beck, Deva, and Beck, James
The Pleasure Connection:
How Endorphins Affect Our Health and Happiness
1. Endorphins   2. Brain Chemistry
3. Science and philosophy   4. Holistic medicine
I. Title
         QP553B43   1987   87-60379
ISBN 0-9617972-0-7

Printed In The United States Of America
By KNI Inc., Anaheim, California
Cover painting by Jonathan Wiltshire
Cover photograph by Michael Kellerman

2 3 4 5 6 7 8 9 0

Dedicated to

Our family—parents, sisters, brothers, and friends. Each of you knows who you are and how your encouragement kept us at the task of finally bringing forth this book. We recognize and salute your love and focus upon life's emerging quality. Special appreciation to Flower A. Newhouse whose teachings and guidance have sown the seeds of these ideas.

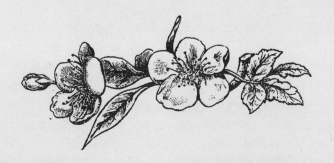

— Acknowledgments —

We wish to thank all the Endorphin research-ers—we've learned so much from you in the course of our studies—Dr. Huda Akil, Dr. Philip A. Berger, Dr. Floyd E. Bloom, Dr. Avram Goldstein, Dr. Roger Guillimen, Dr. John Hughes, Dr. Hans Kosterlitz, Dr. Choh Hao Li, Dr. Candace Pert, Dr. Eric J. Simon, Dr. Lars Terenius, all their associates, and the many others whom we have referenced throughout the text. In a very real way, we feel we know you and tru-ly appreciate your efforts. Your research has enlight-ened the world with possibilities.

We also wish to thank some holistic, body/mind experts and forerunners who helped us to mold our own consciousness along the way—Dr. Fritjof Capra, Norman Cousins, Dr. Marian Diamond, Dr. Neil Fi-ore, Dr. Elisabeth Kubler-Ross, Dr. Robert Ornstein, Dr. Kenneth Pelletier, Dr. Karl Pribram, Dr. Ilya Pri-gogine, Dr. C. Norman Shealy, Dr. Hans Selye, Dr. Carl O. and Stephanie-Matthews Simonton, and Dr. David Sobel. We've attended your workshops, read your books, and learned from your ideas.

Of course, we wish to thank our computer con-sultant, Grant Hulbert, and our editor, Ruth Stock-ton—you encouraged and assisted us through seem-ingly endless revisions to achieve a finished product.

— Foreword —

The most exciting research in science and medicine in the last 30 years, at least, is involved with those miraculous little short chains of amino acid called enkephalins, of which beta-endorphin has received the most attention to date. Most of us believe that we are in the very earliest stages of unraveling this fascinating story of neurotransmitters, and, certainly, each year, more outstandingly useful information arises. *THE PLEASURE CONNECTION* is the best summary to date of this fascinating work. Certainly, every American needs to be aware of the many implications, well-documented and described herein. Even though written for the lay public, many physicians and scientists who are not well acquainted with the endorphin story will find this book most useful. It contains a real encyclopedia of references to the growing literature relating to endorphins and enkephalins. I commend the authors on their very readable and informative presentation.

C. Norman Shealy, M.D., Ph.D.

— Contents —

Contents

Contents

— *Introduction* —

*W*hat do you know about Endorphins? If you're a runner, you've probably experienced runner's "high" and know that Endorphins create euphoria. You might have learned, from a newspaper or magazine article, that Endorphins are the body's own natural biochemical painkillers.

Some Endorphins are known to be hundreds of times more powerful than morphine, and just like morphine, Endorphins can have addictive side effects. Indeed, narcotics like heroin and morphine are, themselves, addictive because their chemistry is similar to our natural Endorphin biochemistry.

Endorphins are triggered by stimulus, stress, and sometimes, even our over-stress responses to the demands of daily life. Because of this, and their own powerful addictive potential, Endorphins now are implicated in the mysteries of heart disease, smoking, alcoholism, depression, arthritis, ulcers, and burnout—some well-known maladies of our stressful times.

But Endorphins are more than biochemicals of stress and harmful addictions. When you are most joyful, Endorphins are flowing. When you feel a chill of gladness down your spine, Endorphins are there. During your deepest happiness—your most meaningful experiences—Endorphins are flowing to enrich your life—to etch these images into your fondest memories. Even as you read these words, Endorphins are circulating throughout your body—an integral part of the bio-electrical flow we call life.

Biochemical research has exploded since Endorphins were discovered over a decade ago. The result? We now have much data about Endorphins—information which points to a fundamental change in scientific concepts about the mind, the body, and how they work together through *bio-electricity* to influence both our health and our happiness.

In a parallel trend, scientists are also expanding our limited notions about disease. This research represents a shift in focus—from the idea of simply coping with and managing disease to a *desire* to maintain optimum well-being.

This trend of consciousness has been termed many things, from stress management, and life extension, to holistic health. It reflects the awareness that all of us are responsible, in great part, for our own health and happiness. Within this view, the *quality* of living is emphasized—physically, mentally, emotionally, and even spiritually.

Have you ever wondered how your mind and brain work together to influence your body? Common sense about everyday encounters helps us to have the perspective that in some way, not completely known, our minds affect our bodies and vice versa. Deep within, you know that there is a connection—but how?

As nurses, we have asked these very questions ourselves. When we learned of Endorphin discoveries, we wondered if this new information would be useful—to help us understand more about ourselves—to help us have a better concept about the connection between the mind's happiness and the body's health.

While we were asking these questions and developing ideas for this book, we were also working as caregivers in traditional medical settings—interacting with people and their needs. As nurses, we are often required to keep an overview of a ward full of patients. Watching on a minute-to-minute basis, throughout a day, a week, or sometimes for months, we see the ebb and flow of disease, sometimes even when the flow of disease ends and health begins. Based on first-hand observations, we have developed an awareness about the flow of recovery and the maintenance of health. We have asked ourselves, will this person regain health? If not, why not? And, what can we do to intercede and help to maximize recovery and sustain well-being? How does Endorphin information apply to this or that situation?

For example, we've observed that some people, even when they're ill, seem to have an extraordinary attitude that significantly enhances their returning health and the very quality of life around them. Other persons "fail to thrive," even when their troubles or illnesses do not seem life-threatening.

We have also learned that pain is subjective and that the rate of recovery is an individual process. We have noted that such nebulous factors as thought, emotions, belief, and attitudes, with their corresponding behavior, are all important clues within the mystery of a healing environment. The knowledge of Endorphins has shed much light on these impressions.

As both nurses and teachers, we have used the combination of our trained observations and our knowledge of Endorphin research to communicate the principles of health. We have found that a knowledgeable explanation from a supportive caregiver becomes as much of a tool as the stethoscope or syringe—an important foundation for ongoing therapy, whatever it may be. When the mind understands and believes, the body is better able to flow toward healing or a resolution of conflict.

As we shall see, the explorations of this book will increase our knowledge about Endorphins—help us to solve our own mind/body puzzles and how we, ourselves, might constructively influence the quality of our lives. We will be exploring how the ebb and flow of Endorphins can correlate with the ebb and flow of our moods and feelings, thoughts, and behavior—as well as the maintenance of our bodies. We will explore how to consciously affect this process—improving our biochemical potential for health and happiness.

In constructing these ideas, we have synthesized experiments, studies, and a broad range of theories into a simple, yet meaningful, format. We have decided to keep our style conversational and contemplative. This choice is made to encourage a reading which helps the reader to understand beyond a memorization of textbook content. We, as authors, will try to present information, asking you, the reader, what you think about a concept. Can you correlate these ideas with your experience? Can you apply what you are learning to your lifestyle choices? If so, we will have mobilized your sense of integrating and synthesizing what you are learning into your own understanding—your own wisdom.

Throughout the book, we will be taking imaginary journeys which are intended to be like field trips where you, as reader, can envision and thus experience examples of what we are observing and learning. Sometimes we will encourage you to draw upon your own experience, sometimes to image an idea you may not have considered before.

At the end of each chapter, you'll find some **How-To Explorations**. Through these suggestions, we hope to provide a bridge that connects you and your life with the challenging, sometimes overwhelming, but fascinating, Endorphin discoveries. You will notice that we are encouraging you to broaden your horizons and assist your discoveries of a new world—where you can begin, or renew, a self-awareness about how the inner aspect of yourself influences your physical state of health. And, based upon these ongoing insights, you might then act upon what you have learned to grow creatively—to live your life with a fuller measure of health, happiness, and indeed, well-being.

If you are involved with helping others in any way, either personally or professionally, we hope that you will be able to formulate your own ideas about how Endorphin information applies to the people you serve. As you use these explorations, your "helping" can become more effective. This book is designed to assist you in applying your emerging understanding of health and well-being to your own life and the lives of the people you touch.

As lovers of life, we hope to bring you joy— elevating the topic of Endorphins far beyond the dusty files of scientific abstracts and into a creative celebration of the best that life has to offer. We hope that this book will bring new meaning to your awareness of life and living—leading you to the shores of a new reality.

Deva Beck, R.N., and James Beck, R.N.
March, 1987

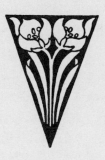

It seems that knowledge gained from viewing old problems from new perspectives can have a profound effect upon the formulation of innovative solutions.   *—Kenneth Pelletier, Ph.D.*

— One —

The Ecology Of Well-Being

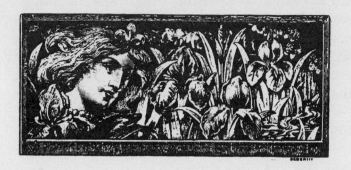

*H*ave you ever found yourself longing for the joy of life? Deep within, you sense the promise of life's meaning and fulfillment. These feelings often arrive suddenly, and seemingly out of nowhere. Exhilaration rises to an overflowing sense of happiness. You tingle with pleasure. A thrill of aliveness cascades down your spine. An inner contentment floods the emotions and mind, creating that mysterious in-ner wholeness known as *euphoria*.

You may be aware that this euphoria arrives because of an event or experience, such as taking a risk, falling in love, or achieving your heart's desire. But, this sense of happiness does not depend necessarily upon an external environment. It can oc-

cur as you remember, or anticipate, something special. This quality of well-being can even touch us
without any apparent cause—for instance, during
a quiet time or moment of still awareness.

Yet, many of us find that, from moment to moment, and day to day, this euphoric experience continues to elude us. Sometimes, even when we have
already achieved yesterday's desires, we still find ourselves longing for that same elusive sense of happiness and well-being. Through research, past and present, we now know that this sensation of well-being
arises from biochemical processes occurring within
the body. In fact, literally all of our physical experiences, and even our thoughts and feelings, are
by-products of this interactive biochemical mix. But
we are not simply by-products of our internal
biochemistry. Like the taste of a soup which can be
influenced by various choices of seasonings—salt,
pepper, or garlic—our internal biochemistry is, in
turn, influenced by our choices, perceptions, feelings,
thoughts, and even attitudes, and beliefs. Together,
all of these influence the quality of our living.

Within this mix of biochemistry, a special family
known as *Enkephalins*, and more commonly called
Endorphins, has recently been discovered. If you
have heard of Endorphins, you may know something of how this amazing finding adds to what is
already known about the mind, the body, and the
mind/body connection. Perhaps you know that the
body can create its own pain relief, or that a runner's "high" comes from these euphoric biochemicals that flood the body. In some instances, Endor-

phins create euphoric pain relief that is several hundred times more powerful than addictive narcotics.

Endorphins create euphoria and pain relief by acting as biochemical messengers, enhancing or diminishing our cells' capability to communicate with one another, storing and sending information within our brains and throughout our bodies.

Although Endorphins are only a few of the many known bodily biochemicals, they are perhaps one of the most significant discoveries of our time—an important connecting link between the mind and the body, and the maintenance of our health and life. Through their inherent capability to create euphoria and relieve pain, Endorphins reinforce or diminish the choices we make every day. In turn, these choices influence our biochemical responses, affecting future choices and events, and our ongoing interaction with life. Responding to these choices our bodies biochemically compensate to maintain the balance in which our potential for health and well-being is optimized.

However, the choices we make in response to life can create internal conflict or stress. If this stress is excessive, it may enhance other predisposing factors like age or genetic weak links to outweigh our ability to adapt or maintain balance. Then "dis-ease" and distress are likely to occur.

For example, if physical, emotional, and mental choices reinforce our need to overeat, and not to exercise, we can become overweight, and even obese. In addition, if we choose to experience a highly stressful life, these factors can combine to increase our risks for heart disease. With each conscious or unconscious choice we make, we enhance or diminish our potential for disease or health, despair or well-being.

Exploring the Cycles of Nature

To illustrate the body's balance toward health and well-being, we can envision one of the balancing cycles within nature. Imagine a high mountain scene where snow-covered peaks harbor a still lake. Once there, walk along the gravel at the low water's edge. In the chilling air, notice that the season will soon change, bringing rain and snow to refill this mountain reservoir.

We can think of the brain to be like our analogy of a mountain reservoir, awaiting the flow of water's precipitation to restore its biochemical life. Like land without water, the brain without this flowing biochemistry would be like a mountain wasteland. In fact, the brain is a biochemical reservoir which harbors the flow of energy we call living. It maintains the ecology of well-being—sustaining physical, mental, and emotional events, and then reflecting these events through biochemical responses which flow from the mountain of the brain into the valleys of the body below.

Picture a cascading waterfall spilling from a mountain lake. This analogy helps us to understand the flow of biochemicals in the body. The brain's hypothalamus, or master gland, is like a whirlpool of energy within the brain's reservoir. Its headwaters begin hormonal, bio-electrical currents flowing into the body—like the rivers flow upon the earth—sustaining the body, stimulating growth and regeneration. Spreading into the lowlands of the body, hormonal and bio-electrical tides are necessary for the maintenance of health and life. Endorphins are now known to be included within these bio-electrical cascades.

Continuing with our analogy, the mountain reservoir is not its own source of water. The lake's primary water source comes from the sea. Neither does the source of our biochemical flow come from the mountains of the brain, itself. Inflow comes to the brain through our five senses, which give us information about the sea of energy which surrounds us. Just as the sea reaches a mountain through evaporation of water and condensation of snow and rain, energy is bio-electrically transmitted through our five senses to the mountain reservoir of the brain, the biochemical processor of our awareness and consciousness.

We can take our nature analogy yet a step further to understand that the body is like an eco-system. Within the cycles of nature, we have come to realize the concept of ecology. If we pollute any part of nature's systems, our ecological balance will be adversely affected. For example, when noxious gas is emitted into the air, rainfall becomes acidic. And then, when acid rain pours into high mountain lakes, the chemistry of ground water changes to affect adversely the survival of lakes and forests, and even entire food chains. So it is with the body—

11

noxious stimuli from physical, mental, and even emotional origins, become biochemical contaminants which will, in due course, adversely affect the overall condition of life.

Discovering the Brain/Mind Connection

In fact, the brain is like a forest composed of billions of branching cells called *neurons*. Neurons are unique because unlike any other cells inside our bodies—they are designed with a tree-like branching system. These branches are termed *axons* and *dendrites*. Axons are the longer branches, often bundled together—like the limbs of a tree—to form what we know to be nerve tracts. Dendrites are shorter and branch at the ends of each axon, just within reach of one another, like the twigs and leaves within the dense tree's foliage. In yet a larger view of this analogy, these branching, intertwining axons and dendrites function together to form a living structure connecting the dense brain foliage through the spinal-cord trunk to roots throughout every part of the body.

Along this network, Endorphins function as communicators, messengers of euphoria, pain relief, and—as we shall see—messengers of the ecological balance of our ongoing health and well-being.

Our neurons are units of communication, like telephone lines, which both receive and transmit impulses through the bio-electrical pathways of axons and dendrites. Our axons are like the heavier telecommunication lines that form nerve tracts traveling long distances. Our dendrites resemble the larger number of smaller lines communicating short distances, as between local homes and businesses.

As you envision these cells and their axons and dendrites, you will notice a seeming density of intertwining structures. Now, bring your field of vision closer so that you can see a slight space appearing between the ends of two dendrites, as they meet each other.

Here, between dendrite and dendrite, a flash of energy occurs. This flash is called a *synapse*. One synaptic flash can be envisioned to be like a single flare within a fireworks display. Each synapse joins with other synaptic flashes to release Endorphins and other biochemicals, igniting the brain's bio-electrical processes, occurring in an ever-ongoing cycle. Imagine trillions of synaptic flashes combining simultaneously to fill the brain and nervous system with infinite bursts of communicating energy.

Remembering our telephone analogy, we note that each synapse acts like an electrical transformer station, enhancing or diminishing biochemical messages traveling along axon and dendrite lines. Responding to sensory messages from the world around us, an ongoing balance of Endorphins is released from these synapses to influence the power of these messages for our health, our experience, and even our consciousness.

At this level of synapses, the brain and its cellular communication become easier to understand. Yet, a connection between the brain's world of dendrite and synapse still seems remote from the mind's conscious ability to influence these same synapses. However, we do affect these biochemical responses every day. We choose and eat food which delivers carbohydrates, glucose, and protein to our biochemical flow. We can also choose to exercise so that these substances can be more effectively synthesized. When we practice these choices well, the flow of our health and well-being reflects this wisdom.

Mental and emotional choices play a significant role in this same biochemical fine tuning of the balance of health. As a simple example, at the mere thought of food, the pancreas secretes insulin for the synthesis of glucose. Just thinking of eating triggers a physical response because mental activity is a biochemical flow of synaptic energy through the brain.

The decathalon gold medalist Bruce Jenner applied this same knowledge to his abilities and success. In addition to arduous physical practice toward his Olympic goals, Bruce Jenner spent time mentally envisioning his physical routines. His concentration focused on imaging the feel or sensation of moving through his practice perfectly. In this way, Bruce Jenner combined mental and physical triggers of a biochemical flow toward his victory.

These examples give us an important hint about how we can and do apply our energies toward triggering a health-giving biochemical flow of Endorphins. For now, let's consider one of the most popular ways to trigger Endorphins—through the stress of physical exercise or feats of endurance. In one laboratory study, both athletes and non-athletes were tested. Their Endorphin levels were reviewed and found to rise significantly as a result of increased exercise.

Running, when pushed to an extreme, just happens to be stressful to the body. Many researchers now believe that it is this additional *stress* of strenuous exercise, rather than the running itself, which triggers the euphoria of Endorphins. It is this stress induced euphoria that gives us a clue about Endorphin flow. When joggers become acclimated to their running routines, they no longer experience the same Endorphin "high" as before. They need to create greater stress for themselves by running faster and or longer to achieve their desire for that feeling. This adaptation problem can also be experienced when these same individuals cannot run. Upon stopping a certain established routine for some reason, many runners notice a change in their general health status. They report a sense of sluggishness and slight irritability, as though they had become dependent upon strenuous exercise to feel good. They think less clearly and are even more susceptible to the latest cold or flu virus. Life becomes more difficult to live. They have become in part—through the mediation of Endorphins—*adapted* to their running routines.

Adaptation and Addiction Clues

But we needn't be joggers to experience stress and adaptation to it. Think about how good it feels to move a stiff leg or arm. After sitting a long while, you then enjoy an opportunity to stand and stretch. You may have noticed that when you have been ill, or confined to one position, you long to get up and move about, having become accustomed to body motion in order to feel good. After recovery, when you are walking again, you feel a rush of euphoria from the activity.

In fact, this slight surge of well-being that is felt while recovering from a short-term illness is similar to the rush of euphoria experienced by runners and other exercise enthusiasts. A recovery period after an illness produces added beneficial stress, as does running an extra mile or lap. In turn, these experiences trigger a euphoric change within the body in response to this stress.

Life is filled with ongoing stressors. Stress can come in the form of changes in our job, home, or relationships. Through our response to these circumstances, we come to adapt to and settle into a routine. When changes occur, we are then forced to adapt again to new situations and surroundings. Without diversity our lives could easily become boring and mundane. Change and our adaptation to change give depth, perspective, and meaning to life.

It would seem that our ability to adapt is a key to our successfully meeting life's ongoing challenges. But adaptation can also turn on us. Our bodies can become overburdened with excessive stress responses. Endorphins play a role in this over-stress response, as well. You'll recall that Endorphins can be hundreds of times more powerful than similar doses of narcotics. Endorphins are powerful and addictive euphoric biochemicals released during stress. We can develop dependence upon—and even addictions to—these internal euphoric biochemicals.

This finding helps us to understand why we can get "high" and addicted to the stressors and challenges of life. We can come to depend upon a stress/adaptation cycle which triggers this euphoric Endorphin process. However, if stress is sustained at high levels for long periods of time, we can become overstressed, losing the body's natural ability to adapt. Yet, at the same time, because of the euphoric properties of Endorphins, we can become addicted to an over-stress response that is detrimental to our health. In fact, this occurs in much the same way that addicts become dependent upon their drugs.

It is helpful here to understand how the addiction process occurs, for it will continue to have many implications as we move through our Endorphin explorations. The cycle of addiction has an established pattern. Over time, the body adapts and develops a tolerance to a small dose of an addictive drug. After the body's natural adaptation process, the same dose that once delivered a feeling of well-being can no longer provide that same pleasure. Then an established tolerance baseline forces the addict to require not only that dose, but also to desire more. To maintain that feeling of well-being over time, higher, more frequent doses must be added, and a vicious cycle begins.

How does this adaptation and tolerance cycle help us understand Endorphins and the delicate balance of health? Let's explore how this tolerance/

dependence cycle occurs. Visualize a cell within your body. Looking closely at this cell, you will discover, as researchers did, a biochemical "keyhole." These keyholes, officially called *receptor sites*, are uniquely designed to receive a special kind of chemical key. A biochemical with that special composition or design would then be the key that would fit the cell's receptor. When this biochemical key and receptor keyhole come together, a dynamic response occurs within the cell. Like a car that requires an ignition key to operate, our cells require biochemical keys to ignite our bodily processes.

Many drugs are also biochemical keys that can fit keyhole receptors in our cells. This is true of the addictive narcotics like heroin, a powerful opium chemical which unlocks a keyhole receptor in our cells. Through this action, we can experience both pain relief and euphoria from narcotics. When someone is hopelessly addicted to the pleasure obtained from heroin or other opium derivatives, a powerful interlocking chemical process occurs inside the addict's cells. This "keyhole" clue leads to an understanding of the underlying nature of addiction. As noted by the early Endorphin researcher Dr. Avram Goldstein, obviously, God did not intend these receptor sites for the exclusive pleasure of heroin addicts. He surmised that because receptor sites exist, then there also must be internal biochemical keys somewhere within the body, itself. Heroin and morphine simply are external copies of another pleasure-inducing biochemical key created inside our bodies.

This essential concept was the impetus which led,

in due course, to the discoveries of the family of internal *keys* called Endorphins. In the past decade, at least twelve distinct substances have been proven to belong to this group of brain biochemicals, now known to have profound, wide-ranging effects upon us.

We now know that Endorphin keys (like the external "copy" called heroin), connect with Endorphin keyholes to create pain relief and euphoria. But, just as significantly, Endorphin keyholes have been found within the brain, spinal cord, and also throughout the body—along the digestive system, upon cells of the pancreas, spleen, kidneys, heart, lungs, reproductive organs, and the immune system. Thus, researchers now believe that Endorphins which fit into these far-reaching keyholes play a comprehensive role in the total maintenance of our health.

This wide range of discovered keyhole clues gives us a hint about the extraordinary Endorphin connection between our sense of happiness and the biochemical ecology of our health and well-being.

Stimulus Becomes Another Key

Knowing about the possibility of Endorphin keyholes even before they were discovered, Dr. Huda Akil, a researcher then at the University of California, Los Angeles, took a landmark approach to Endorphin explorations.

To develop her experiment, Dr. Akil utilized a pain-killing phenomenon which had long remained a mystery to medical observers. For centuries, the use of electrical stimulus—from ancient treatments with electric eels to sophisticated wiring techniques—had often provided amazing pain relief. Dr. Akil wondered if electricity which had been used throughout history to kill pain, somehow created the internal chemical key and thus produced a diminished response to pain. To probe this mystery, she decided to test a well-known chemical antidote called *naloxone*.

Naloxone is a drug used as an emergency antidote for heroin and morphine overdose. Naloxone literally reverses the effect of opiate-induced coma, dramatically awakening a slumbering addict. (This drug even reverses heroin's euphoria, making dependent persons irritable, sometimes hostile and combative.)

In previous experiments, Dr. Akil already had used naloxone as an antidote for morphine. Using morphine to provide pain relief for her laboratory animals, Dr. Akil then reversed this effect with doses of naloxone. As expected, the use of naloxone returned the pain which morphine had relieved. Then she asked a question which would result in a landmark clue. Would naloxone also reverse the pain relief mysteriously induced by electrical stimulus?

Just as she previously had given morphine to reduce pain, Dr. Akil applied measured electrical stimulus into the brain of one of her rats. As before, this dose of electricity equaled morphine relief. Naloxone was then given to her electrically stimulated animal. Immediately, the antidote reversed the relief gained from electricity. Once again, Dr. Akil's subject showed quicker symptoms of pain.

Every rat tested exhibited the same result. The morphine antidote, naloxone, had likewise reversed the pain-killing effect of electricity. Thus, naloxone must have indeed reversed the effect of a previously unknown, but powerful, internal pain-killing biochemical. Naturally occurring brain biochemicals, soon to be identified as Endorphins, had somehow been induced by the stimulus of electricity.

Dr. Akil's study of electrically stimulated pain relief, with corresponding naloxone reversal, did more than imply the actions of Endorphins. Her experiment was itself a key to the unlocking of an Endorphin door for us.

Dr. Akil's observations clarify the fact that electrical stimulus actually modifies the subtle mix of biochemicals within our bodies. With these observations in mind, let's return to our earlier mountain imagery. You'll recall that the mountain was not its own source of water. The mountain required a life-sustaining inflow of energy from the sea in the form of condensation, rain, and snow. Our five senses give our brains similar life-sustaining inflows of bio-electrical energy. A major ongoing source of brain stimulus creates an environment conducive to life, through the bio-electrical pathways of our five senses.

We know that our eyes see images, that our ears hear sounds. But images and sounds are translated into bio-electrical messages that flow as electrical stimuli to our brains. Through touch, we learn electrical information about varieties of texture—rough, smooth, hard, and soft. Similarly, taste and smell, closely interconnecting sensory processes, receive and send bio-electrical stimuli from taste buds and olfactory nerve endings. In fact, we become interactive with life through this same electrical stimulus of our sensory awareness.

As you would already expect, the flow of Endorphins is the triggered result of these five sensory stimuli. Powerful pain relievers and biochemicals of euphoria play primary roles in all of these interactive sensory processes. For example, Endorphins are involved in the singing of birds and the schooling of fish. In fact, Endorphin keyholes have been discovered on the sensory cells of many animals. Even the one-celled protozoan owns Endorphin keyholes.

Sensory awareness is an intricate, ongoing, and interactive process responsible for every experience throughout life. But, our senses give us far more than information about the outside world. Our five senses combine with our sensations of pleasure and pain, intertwined by the flow of Endorphins. Acting as messengers of both sensory stimulus and pleasure, Endorphins are bio-electrical messengers which influence the way we perceive our environment.

A Holographic Brain/Mind

To understand how sensory stimulus is integrated into our perceptions of reality and our own individual sense of happiness and well-being, imagine that you are sitting in a comfortable chair. Your chair is placed exactly between two stereo speakers. You know this audio experience well. If two stereo speakers are placed just so, your favorite music no longer seems to originate from the speakers, themselves. Indeed, music then floods the room, seeming to come from all places, simultaneously. This integration of sound is what sound specialists call *phase relationship*.

Through our five sensory electrical pathways, a similar phase relationship is achieved. Dr. Karl Pribram, a brain surgeon and researcher at Stanford University, has conceived of a brain theory that incorporates this phase-relationship analogy. During his long career, Dr. Pribram began to make new and more comprehensive observations about brain processes. Prior to Dr. Pribram's ideas, the brain was thought to be composed simply of different anatomical areas. In this earlier theory, each brain part was a separate entity, and each had its own distinct function, separate from the others.

In our analogy, the different, distinct brain locations are like the different, individual stereo speakers. The energy that flows through each speaker—in this case, the music—becomes a synthesized experience of sound. Likewise, Dr. Pribram's expanded view of brain processes demonstrates that, although there are separate, specialized brain locations, all are channels of brain energy that become synthesized into unified experiences.

While searching for his own analogy to explain his observations, Dr. Pribram learned of a specialized kind of photography called *holography*. This is a form of lensless, three-dimensional photography utilizing laser beams to record the image. You may have heard of holography as the technology used in the movie *Star Wars* to achieve the special effect of Princess Leia's three-dimensional image projected by R2-D2. Holographs are also now being incorporated on the face of credit cards to make them more difficult to counterfeit. The ghostly images found in the Haunted House at Disneyland are also holographic.

From his research into holographs Dr. Pribram developed a theory about the *holographic brain*, explaining how holographic energy is similar to the brain's electrical capability to experience a unified five-sensory awareness.

As information is biochemically passed through our five senses and back to the brain, this electrical energy becomes like the laser beams in holography. The brain's five-dimensional reality becomes analogous to a three-dimensional hologram. The holographic brain synthesizes five simultaneous electrical stimuli in the same integrated, phase relationship we have already explored. Environmental stimuli, laser-like energy sources, impact their information upon us by interacting with the living holograms that create our brain/mind processes, synthesizing the constant inflow of brain bio-electricity.

In Dr. Pribram's theory, our brains are simply and majestically like screens which suspend the holograms of our minds. Dr. Pribram's theory suggests that brain processes, like holography, are capable of changing our five-sensory pathway into the integrated pictures we call reality. But, our brains are not merely passive receptors of these holographic images. Our bio-electrical mental and emotional processes also play active roles in our conscious and unconscious choices, acting like editors of the holographic movies of our experience.

Through this sensory network, we filter information through the electrical energies of our minds and emotions, accept what we need to perceive, and reject what is perceived as irrelevant, thereby defining our ongoing realities. In these ways we physically and mentally synthesize all incoming stimuli that act upon our senses, into one five-sensory phase-relationship.

Furthermore, we maintain memories of all past stimuli, both conscious and unconscious. Through these bio-electrical stimuli, Endorphins play a significant role in the formation and retention of memory.

Perhaps you can recall a vital memory, one carrying such an energy impact upon you that it remains much clearer or more meaningful to you than even your present experience. For instance, you might have noticed that a particular smell may instantly return a distant memory to you; it has remained fully alive, stored away within your brain. Endorphins are implicated in both the biochemical return of memory and the bio-electrical sense of smell. Thus, it is easy to understand how the aroma of baking bread could transmit you electrically to a replay of a childhood experience. Likewise, the smell of burning rubber might bring to mind the scene of an automobile accident. These are examples of how a complete holographic image can be stored within one sensory awareness.

These are holographic visions, encoded throughout your brain by powerful biochemicals which have etched a meaningful five-sensory image or replay into your memory. These memory holograms interact with present sensory electrical input to modify and define our own unique perceptions and reactions, which we each then call reality. Remember, these same biochemical processes, which include Endorphins, are important brain/mind connections influencing our health and well-being.

Returning once again to Dr. Pribram's observations, we can achieve a unified understanding of our brains. Dr. Pribram noted another resemblance between the brain and holograms—every small energy cell of the brain reflects a unique miniature version of the whole brain, itself. This concept is akin to the phenomenon we can observe on a damp, sunlit morning. Each small dewdrop becomes a prism reflecting a unique miniature version of the sun.

Carrying this idea further, imagine a densely flowered tree standing in the bright sunlight. The tree's structure recalls our earlier reviews of the brain's tree-like branching system. Reaching from the farthest edges of the brain, through the microscopic branchings of axons and dendrites, our brains make a limb-like connection down through the spinal trunk to communicate even with the dendrite roots in our fingers and toes.

In our early-morning scene, this imagined tree

would glisten with sun-reflected biochemical dew. Picture this tree's structure transformed into a bright sphere, fully alight and rainbow-colored with prism dewdrops. There is a splendor about our vision because the tree seems vitally alive.

Looking closer, we see that each dewdrop reflects the tree around it, becoming a bright sphere within a sphere. Every small nerve cell or energy "dewdrop" of the brain seems to *reflect* a unique miniature version of the whole brain. Seeming to have a life of its own, each dewdrop radiates a poised and beautiful potential.

Again remembering Dr. Pribram's concepts, we can envision these millions of brain cells within the brain's sphere to look something like our resplendent tree. Each shining dewdrop is akin to the energy essence of a cell, the tree a sphere of energy representing the brain, itself. We can consider our sphere of energy as being both the process of brain bio-electricity and the process for the energies of our minds and emotions.

Longing for a Quick Fix

Endorphins are some of the biochemicals ignited through trillions of synaptic flashes—the flow of these brain/mind processes. Endorphin researchers, who have painstakingly isolated these incredibly tiny biochemicals which have so much power to impact upon our life's experience, tell us that Endorphins are not only small—they are unbelievably short-lived! The lives of many Endorphins are measured in brief moments of time. From one second to the next, our biochemical flow continues on. From the perspective of this tiny yet all-pervading reality, our brains do not channel the same biochemical and electrical river experienced a moment ago. Nor are we what we will soon become.

Have you ever felt a fleeting sense of bliss? It happens like a slight mist evaporating upon your face—so brief that before you are more than half aware, it has disappeared, a phantom feeling, a moment vanished even as you perceived it and defined its meaning. This phantom is a good example of the quick bliss which tiny Endorphins can bring to us.

You might have felt this joy while listening to a glorious birdsong, smelling a flower's fragrance, or watching a beautiful sunset. Thrill-seekers press the throttle of this feeling, forcing the possible risk to their lives to maintain that phantom bliss. Painters, sculptors, dancers, musicians, and poets—artisans of all kinds—catch glimpses of this bliss in their work to create color, form, rhythm, and sound. Mothers know it in bonding with their children.

Those who are in love with life seem to enjoy a never-ending flow of this same kind of experience. This fleeting, yet potent, mist of feeling seems to promise meaning in our lives, a promise that is sometimes fulfilled.

When we are troubled, we long for a sense of peace and ease. Perhaps this is because we have known the flow of joy, and somehow, through a quick change of brain biochemistry, we now perceive this same joy to be residing far from us. Whether we are troubled and in a state of yearning or we are exuberantly "high," we are like the addict, longing for a quick "fix." A momentary flash of biochemical euphoria and the wonderful feeling is gone. And in our darkness we long for it again.

❋ ❋ ❋

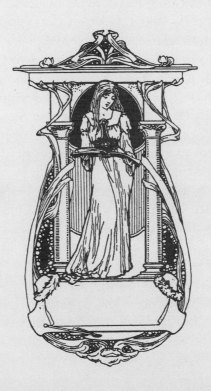

HOW-TO EXPLORATIONS TO TRY

—For Endorphin clues in your own body, consider the times you have been "high" on physical activity. Did you achieve this feeling after an increase in your activity level? What sensations did you feel at that time? Did this change improve your outlook on life? Or vice versa? When your activity level is decreased, do you feel depressed, sluggish, or "out of sorts" with the world?

—Recall if you have ever become addicted to stress, such that an over-stress response became detrimental to your health? Have you ever pushed yourself too hard—trying to solve a problem—finding that your own push response was blocking the solution? Have you ever enjoyed working overtime, or staying up late to work on a project only to find the next day that you are run down, susceptible to illness, or less capable of coping with life stressors? Record your impressions.

—Return to your earlier imagery of the densely flowering tree alight with sun-reflected dew. Each dewdrop is one neuron—poised and ready to reflect an awareness that combines present stimulus with all your previous experiences, to give you a holographic image of your ongoing reality. What stimulus or past experiences have shaped your significant holographic images of today? Are these images comfortable for you—or are there some you would like to change?

Ecology Of Well-Being

—Notice what sensory stimulus makes you feel good, and expand these feelings by broadening your experiences to include new sensory awareness. While outdoors, pay attention to sounds and smells that give you pleasure. Often, we forget to use these potent sources of stimulus, not realizing our potential capability to experience life fully.

—Recall a vivid memory of a past experience and notice the power of that memory toward physical responses in your body. Ask yourself if your present choices of behavior or response to life are based on previous impressions that are no longer valid or applicable to present conditions. Take note of these impressions.

—As Bruce Jenner did, use mental imagery to "feel" your body move through one of your physical experiences. If you are refining a physical technique in sports, dancing, or recreation, use imagery to improve your performance. This technique can also be used in perfecting a new mental attitude or changing an emotional belief.

—To improve your understanding of how your brain biochemistry works, take your imagination down to a microscopic level. Pretend that you can watch synapses flash as they occur between two dendrites—the ongoing release of energy that can be likened to a fireworks display. Each flare is one synapse. But now, envision the display, bright with millions of synaptic flares. As you watch these bursts of energy, identify one color, imagining that you can watch the flow of your own Endorphins. See them burst in and amongst the other flares to cascade through the network of dendrites, axons, and nerve tracts within your body. Now, as you breathe deeply, try to feel your Endorphins flowing to help you feel happy—both relaxed and alert, from within your own natural biochemistry.

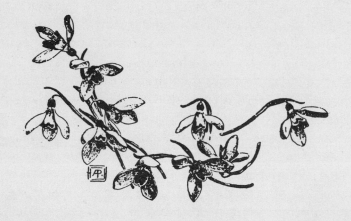

To ward off disease or recover health, men as a rule find it easier to depend on healers than to attempt the more difficult task of living wisely.
　　　　　　　　　　　　　　　　　—Rene Dubos

— Two —

Seeking A Delicate Balance

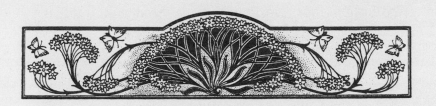

$\mathcal{P}$owerful, euphoric, pain-killing Endorphins, flowing through our brains' biochemistry, a communicating network throughout our bodies with the potential to keep us healthy, pain-free, and even happy—then, why is it not always so? If the biochemical potential for happiness is there within us, why isn't it always a biochemical reality?

A thorny question arises. If these biochemicals of happiness, called Endorphins, exist, why then do we endure so much pain and suffering? What triggers an Endorphin response? What would make it stop, or not begin at all? If Endorphins are such potent pain-killers, where are they when we need relief most? When we endure pain, why wouldn't the body's own pain-killing mechanism also respond to any and every pain we know, to keep us always free of suffering, anxiety, and discontent? These questions bring us to the core of our study of Endorphins. Through these questions, we can begin exploring Endorphin research to seek some basic answers for ourselves.

To understand Endorphins better and our relationship to them, we need to return to the study of our incredible brains, which harbor much of the Endorphin environment. It is here, within the vast complexity of brain processes, that many of the body's regulatory biochemicals are created. Scientists are beginning to understand that the brain functions through an ongoing, fluctuating flow of biochemical and electrical events. In order that we might better understand this process within a larger context, let's consider a river flowing within the cycles of nature.

Exploring Nature's Interdependent Balance

Imagine that we journey to a canyon where desert and mountains meet. Once there, we walk along a dry creek bed. With the season's change, the rushing water will soon flood this parched gully, becoming a turbulent river bringing life to the desert.

Now we can hear a torrent tumbling down upon the rocks below and watch the surging flow of water as it rushes by. We can pick our way along its banks for awhile. This experience is a participation in an ongoing event that continues for as long as the water flows.

A Delicate Balance

When we think of the brain, itself, in relation to Endorphin action, we can consider it to be like a dry creek bed. The brain is a similar channel, awaiting a river of biochemical events. This brain river is a process, an ever-changing flow of energy that we recognize as our existence, the fact of our living. From this image, we can gain a broadened perspective that helps us to understand more about Endorphin activity.

Returning to our imagery—we have discovered a canyon within the mountain peaks where melting snows run to quench a desert thirst. Among these tumbled boulders lies the potential for drought or oasis, as well as for flash floods. The force of the flow and the delicate balance of nature determine the river's nourishment or devastation.

Within our own delicate flow of brain biochemistry, balanced or imbalanced, lies the potential for our health or disease. The brain's constant, life-giving river of biochemicals runs to keep us alive and well when it is functioning as it should. If not, diseased conditions of "drought" or "flood" may begin.

In this canyon setting, we could choose to imagine any type of season and corresponding river flow. If we have chosen summer, there would still be a moderate flow of water, dwarfed beside the huge boulders in the river. Sounds would be so gentle in the quiet canyon that we might have to sit very still to hear them well. We'll place ourselves upon a comfortable rock in the cool shade and consider life's ease. So relaxed, we could contemplate or doze, wondering why we had ever worried or felt alarm. If life has seemed stressful to us, the challenges have trickled away downstream, far removed from this present moment. We perceive that the world seems wonderful. Within our bodies, a balance of biochemicals corresponds with our mood and consciousness.

We are still, our heartbeats are steady and quiet. We breathe deeply, slowly. If we have just enjoyed a picnic, we can notice that the warmth within our bodies is almost a happy feeling as digestive processes easily take the food we've eaten and turn it into nourishment for our cells.

This biochemical balance is called the *parasympathetic response*, or the body's capability to relax. Throughout the brain and nervous system, biochemicals of relaxation can predominate, giving our bodies the calm and rest they need for life's maintenance. Endorphins are known to be involved in the lowering of blood pressure, the slowing of heart rate, the digestive processes, the relaxation of muscles, the freedom from pain, the sense of euphoric consciousness. They may indeed be the body's intrinsic tranquilizers. The parasympathetic response also predominates when our bodies need repair from illness or injury.

As we rest after our picnic, the vessels in our bloodstream dilate, our blood circulation improves. All sense of pain and tension has vanished from our awareness. Our consciousness is at ease, euphoric. The river runs quiet beside our resting place and we find ourselves asleep, bathed in the dappled sunlight.

Then, autumn arrives and the air is even more

still. The water level has decreased, diminished to a few standing pools in the rocks, nearby. The sense of life and activity is at a low ebb. Leaves hover, still, with no breeze to blow them. Wild life no longer comes to drink, for the pools have been standing too long without fresh input.

We'll imagine that we have slept deeply, lying still far too long. Perhaps we can feel a sense of immense lethargy, no longer vital, as though we too have stagnated. No fresh flow of activity has come to nourish our lives. This sensation may make us feel engulfed in depression, numb to sensation, and without a sense of being alive. Parasympathetic biochemicals over-predominate. The prior sense of relaxation has gone too far out of balance.

At this point in our imagery, we may wish to get up, move about, shake the cobwebs from our consciousness, and stimulate our being. At the University of Wisconsin, exercise researchers have noted this response also. A group of psychiatrists, psychologists, and a physical education instructor have developed the use of stimulus therapy—running exercise to improve the mood and motivation of lethargic, depressed persons. This response is, of course, the body's balancing mechanism. Our biochemical longing for stimulus is now just as strong as was a prior relaxation biochemistry urging us to sleep.

Through biochemical longing, we now seek to experience the opposite, active biochemical flow—the *sympathetic response*. Its common name of "fight or flight" describes its actions upon the body. When the sympathetic nervous system is activated by a stressor, we are biochemically assisted to react effectively. Our hearts beat faster, our breathing is more rapid, deeper and easier, and we can think quickly and with clarity. We are prepared bodily and mentally to take on a fight or to run fast, and to make a quick judgment about which is best.

Thus our bodies have a balancing mechanism called the *autonomic nervous system*. Two so-called *branches* of response—parasympathetic and sympathetic, act in seemingly opposite ways. Through this balancing, the parasympathetic and sympathetic responses are dependent upon each other for the regulation of our health.

Endorphins play a role of mediators in intertwining the sympathetic and parasympathetic systems, acting as negotiators toward an ongoing interdependent balance. When one response over-predominates, as in the case of parasympathetic imbalance linked with depression, a stimulus is needed to swing the balance back to a sympathetic response.

As we have learned earlier in this chapter, the stimulus of increased exercise is being used as a therapy for depression. Endorphins are activated by this stimulus. With the push of exercise, the body swings from the over-dominant, parasympathetic mode of depression. The "high" that runners feel when they push themselves beyond their current exercise tolerance is a hint of the role Endorphins play as mediators in this balancing process.

Adapting to the Tides of Stress

Our adaptation to stress is also an example of the balance between parasympathetic and sympathetic responses. This adaptation process has been thoroughly studied and described by the famous stress expert Dr. Hans Selye. According to Dr. Selye's observations, we biochemically respond to stress with a process which allows us to cope with it. When stress occurs for us, our bodies are designed to respond to this onslaught with a progressive series of biochemical changes which maintain the ongoing balance of health.

Observing this adaptation cycle, Dr. Selye developed his stress theories in the 1950s, long before Endorphins were discovered. We now know that stress is a stimulus which can trigger Endorphins. Through the euphoric power of the Endorphin process, we are physically and emotionally assisted to adapt to that stress, again, by maintaining the parasympathetic/sympathetic balance within the body.

In a 1981 issue of *Psychology Today*, Dr. Agu Pert, a pharmacologist at the National Institute for Mental Health, reviews studies which show how Endorphins assist us in adapting to stress. Dr. Pert's article cites numerous studies about the physical stressor of pain, itself. These studies have shown that our bodies respond to painful stimulus by manufacturing Endorphins to provide pain relief and stress adaptation.

Dr. Lars Terenius, an early Endorphin researcher in Uppsala, Sweden, has written a similar review in a recent editorial for the *American Heart Journal*. Dr. Terenius suggests that Endorphins are also involved in the parasympathetic adaptation to the anxiety one feels, perceiving the sympathetic increase of stress factors in his life.

In perhaps the first clearly documented example of euphoric parasympathetic response to stress, Dr. Henry K. Beecher writes of an important observation he made during World War II. During this combat, military physicians who attended the victims noticed a strange phenomenon. Many soldiers who had been severely mutilated by war injuries exhibited a behavior known as *combat euphoria*. While their wounds were being treated, these soldiers remained very calm and peaceful, exhibiting parasympathetic ease. They seemed even happy, as though their serious injuries were of no consequence to them. Although aware of these obvious afflictions, they laughed and joked, rather than feeling the sympathetic response of intense pain and anxiety.

We have seen how the stimulus of combat and other sympathetic stressors seem to trigger a parasympathetic Endorphin response. Could Endorphins be triggered by other kinds of stimuli? At the University of Calgary in Alberta, Canada, researchers have asked that same question. They found that Endorphins are induced by the stimulus of extreme temperature change. You may have tried this same Endorphin experiment many times yourself, noticing that an ice pack can relieve a headache. We now know that the ice pack stimulus induces the flow of pain-killing Endorphins to naturally relieve discomfort. Likewise, heat packs and heating pads are a well-known pain-killing remedy for chronic backache.

In the study at Calgary, the opiate antagonist, naloxone, which we already have learned about in Chapter One, was used to observe biochemical responses to heat and cold. Naloxone was found to block the body's capacity of adaptation to temperature extremes. This finding implies that the Endorphin response, known to be blocked by the naloxone antagonist, is a part of our biochemical ability to adapt to climate.

This research finding of Endorphin-enhanced adaptation to climate extremes leads us to additional interesting research about the role of Endorphins throughout our bodily processes. The hibernation response, clearly a survival mechanism found in many animal living in cold climates, presents a clue about the role of Endorphins. As we have noted from the above findings completed in Alberta, Endorphins are triggered by the stress of extreme cold. In a survival behavior attributed to instinct, bears and other forest mammals eat heavily to store energy against a snow-induced famine. Endorphins are now considered to contribute a biochemical reinforcement for the hibernation instinct.

This information recalls the earlier imagery of a picnic beside a waterfall. As you envisioned that lunch nourishing your body, the parasympathetic response began to relax you and you felt the urge to sleep. Naps and hibernation are two examples of parasympathetic Endorphin responses, one short and the other long.

Remember that eating food often provides a good feeling? In prior eras, when food was not so plentiful, the tendency toward maintaining extra body weight was considered a reserve against famine, a savings account against losses through foul weather and illnesses, such as tuberculosis and plague. People who were heavier had a better chance of living longer. They were the survivors. It is only in recent decades and here, where technology supplies vast food quantities, that obesity seems an extravagance. Only in these times do we consider obesity to be a possible addiction to eating. Would Endorphins be the biochemicals responsible for the survival response of eating well? Is eating potentially addictive because powerful, euphoric, parasympathetic biochemicals reinforce the behavior of taking food?

Since hibernation is an example of the instinctual Endorphin reinforcement to eat heavily and survive, it would be easy to connect the addictive response of Endorphins with a euphoric behavior of overeating. Biochemical euphoria may be correlated with the sense of feeling satisfied, even happy, after a plentiful meal. From this eating-induced euphoria, many respond to their sympathetic sense of stress by overeating. In this way, a survival mechanism can become a maladaptive use of the parasympathetic balance toward coping with stress.

Therefore, it is not surprising that studies indeed

have linked stress-induced overeating with Endorphins. Researchers at the University of Minnesota, in Minneapolis, have suggested that it is the euphoric and pain-killing action of Endorphins which leads to the overuse of food to cope with stress.

At Temple University, Dr. David L. Margules has correlated increased levels of Endorphins with becoming obese in response to stress. In *Psychology Today*, he suggests examples of how this behavior might be treated. Again, the opium antagonist, naloxone, has been utilized. Dr. Margules and his colleagues awakened hibernating hamsters by injecting them with naloxone. If naloxone can reverse a hibernation coma, could it therefore be a treatment for the obesity induced by an Endorphin-addictive appetite overeating?

In several research situations, naloxone has been used to reduce weight gain. Most of these studies have used mice and rats who are genetically obese and inclined to overeat. In comparison to lean animals, these rodents also have higher levels of Endorphins in their blood and pituitary glands. When the genetically heavier animals were given naloxone, they stopped their overeating response. (The same naloxone doses did not affect lean animals.)

Also, one researcher has reported a forty-eight-day trial of naloxone on himself with "impressive" weight loss during that time.

In these examples, we have seen how our bodies respond to sympathetic stress. Through these responses, we develop preferences of behavior, increasing our parasympathetic ability to maintain a balance through a stressful period. We have especially noted that researchers are beginning to show how Endorphins assist these parasympathetic adaptations with their own powerful capacities. Endorphins can help us to adapt, keeping us relaxed, well, and even happy, in times of stress. Endorphins help us increase our potential for survival in a famine condition.

Sometimes, however, Endorphins can help us reinforce coping behavior that creates unwanted side effects. For instance, coping with stress by overeating can lead to obesity.

Adaptation Becomes Maladaptation

The parasympathetic response can over-predominate to become a risk factor as potentially harmful as the original sympathetic stressor, itself. Endorphins play a role in this more ominous form of adaptation. We will refer to this harmful parasympathetic dominance as *maladaptation* and explore how Endorphins also function to assist this response.

You have probably noticed that different people respond to the stress in their lives in different ways. Some persons seem to handle stress well, are less concerned by an initial challenge, less bothered by daily irritations, and remain calmer longer through a lengthy calamity in their lives. It would seem that these individuals have a biochemical design that allows them to endure. Others fit the opposite description. Their "short fuses" are also biochemical.

A Delicate Balance

They seem to lack a natural parasympathetic balance. Little details or changes in routine are sympathetically stressful. They find themselves overwhelmed more often. Their adaptation capacity ends much more quickly, and major stressors devastate them.

In theory, we can imagine a variable Endorphin response which helps to explain differences in stress responses. These differences in stress responses help us to get a good perspective on maladaptation. We already know how important high Endorphin levels are in the relaxation response. Those people who seem to cope well with stress may have more constant and enduring parasympathetic Endorphins to rely upon biochemically. Thus, they would be enabled to relax with consistency. Irritable, highly stressed people may really have a short supply of these same Endorphins or fewer Endorphin receptor sites that would help them to adapt naturally to life. These people, who function on lower levels of biochemical euphoria, could well seek the parasympathetic Endorphin response in a maladaptive way.

For example, imagine an unfortunate person beginning on the road to drug addiction. He is haunted by the promise of freedom from stress with an artificial experience of drugged pleasure. Perhaps this one's life is a prison of difficulties and stress. Within a confinement of over-stress, there may be no new inflow of parasympathetic biochemistry to give this person a sense of possibilities for the natural feeling of being happily relaxed and well. And yet, a biological longing, perhaps an Endorphin depletion, gives this addict a feeling of intense deprivation. The stage is set for an unscrupulous drug supplier to enter and tempt with the artificially induced addictive process.

Let's review briefly what happens next, because the addiction mechanism will help us to understand better how Endorphins play a role in diseases of maladaptation. A starting dose of an addictive drug is begun. This dose is relatively small, just a pinch to make it through the day. It does the job and the world seems better, a bit more tolerable and bearable. When this dose is active, instant relief and happiness are experienced. An artificial flow of euphoria arises.

Remember, we now know that this happens because a drug's action mimics the natural parasympathetic Endorphin "high" induced by the stimulus of increased exercise or stress. Soon, the artificial drug wears off and the sense of depletion, lack of flow, and longing begin again. Within this sad life, there is no generation of stimulus for the river of intrinsic Endorphins to begin flowing; while the addict perceives that the external substance is the only way of triggering a pleasure "high."

Because of longing and corresponding stress, subsequent doses are taken. Perhaps these doses hold as long and well, perhaps they do not. The next dose might be taken sooner or be larger in amount. Whenever the amount and frequency increase, the rising need for artificial relief parallels the dulling, diminishing response of the body's own natural biochemical process. The problem compounds itself as the natural Endorphin response seems to be even more depressed, finally into total depletion and stagnation.

As the addictive cycle continues, longing also continues for more and more of the artificial pleasure. This tolerance/dependence process is easily understood within a drug addiction example. But this maladaption occurs because its sequence is designed within our own naturally occurring Endorphin flow, within the brain's own biochemical river.

It is easy to plug addictive drugs into our theory. In these extreme examples, an addict limits the stimulus/stress response to a substance which limits the body's capability to cope with stress. The drug itself is the only euphoric stress adaptation that an addict may rely upon.

But what about other kinds of addictive responses? We know how addictive the natural Endorphin high can be. Is this Endorphin response somehow involved in the maladaptation of other, more legal and socially acceptable, addictions? Could the cycles of Endorphin flow be responsible for parasympathetic maladaptations that become harmful to our health?

Endorphins, Alcohol, and Nicotine

As you can guess, many researchers have sought to answer this very question. As a result, we have a variety of studies to review. You may have been wondering how the use of alcohol links with the flow of Endorphins. Alcohol is a substance used to imitate the parasympathetic response of ease and relaxation. Alcohol's use can become overuse when someone takes alcohol in order to cope with the anxieties and stressors of the world. Thus, a maladaptive cycle begins an artificial parasympathetic response to stress in a potentially harmful way. Because its immoderate intake is so harmful to our health and our society, the overuse of alcohol may be considered a maladaptation to stress.

Because of the addictive aspect of alcoholic intake, it is not surprising that much study has been developed to link alcoholic mechanisms with the presence or absence of Endorphins in our bodies. When Endorphins were first discovered, researchers were enthusiastic about the possibility that alcohol use might trigger natural Endorphins. Another possibility was that alcohol, itself, might fit the keyhole receptor site, thereby inducing an addiction similar to that of morphine and heroin. These simple answers have not been found. However, a complex chain of biochemical events, which begins with the intake of alcohol, is now receiving considerable Endorphin-research interest.

Researchers throughout the world, in places as divergent as the United States, South America, Australia, and Europe have pursued this study. At the Max-Planck Institute for Psychiatry in Munich, West Germany, the main Endorphin-research thrust has become the connection between Endorphins and the addiction of alcohol.

One line of research has focused upon alcohol

addiction and a corresponding deficiency of Endorphins. At the University of Cagliari in Pavia, Italy, scientists have used experiments to further the idea that chronic alcohol use somehow depletes the body's capability to continue a flow of intrinsic Endorphins. If this is so, they reason, it could be that a hunger or longing for the biochemical euphoria of Endorphins would increase a seeking after the artificial parasympathetic feeling that alcohol provides.

You may also be wondering about another very common maladaptation to stress—the use of nicotine. Indeed, brain researchers have wondered about cigarettes, too. It is well known that cigarette smoking is heavily addictive. People simply feel good when they smoke. It becomes a habit which gives smokers a sense of ease and relaxation. Once again, the natural parasympathetic balance is artifically induced.

Additionally, smokers report that while they are smoking they feel less tired, even quite alert and better able to remember with specific clarity. Often, when we feel relaxed and easy, we also notice drowsiness, our senses are dulled, and we often are engulfed by sleep. But smoking initiates a specialized kind of ease, one which allows the smoker to stay simultaneously alert and relaxed. At this time, nicotine is the only known drug to have this action.

In a 1984 issue of the *Brain/Mind Bulletin*, reports of research about smoking and Endorphins have been published. At the University of Connecticut, Dr. Ovide Pommerleau is tracking the biochemicals which are enhanced with the use of nicotine. Prior to Dr. Pommerleau's work, brain scientists had considered that Endorphins might be involved in the pleasure associated with nicotine use. Dr. Pommerleau's data have shown that increased Endorphin production does indeed correspond with nicotine levels in blood. But his discoveries have continued beyond correlating nicotine use with an increase in Endorphins.

Noting the alertness benefit of smoking, Dr. Pommerleau has also traced an increase in other brain biochemicals. He found that nicotine enhances vasopressin, which assists with memory. He also noted smoking's increase of epinephrine and norepinephrine, which enhance arousal. Dr. Pommerleau has additionally found that nicotine increases levels of dopamine, which was, prior to the discovery of Endorphins, considered to be the brain biochemical of reward.

While this list of brain biochemicals may make cigarette smoking seem more enticing, additional findings show that nicotine is dangerous. It is the stress of smoking which initiates these responses. Sound familiar? We have already learned that stress can be a stimulus to naturally occurring pleasure biochemicals. As the cycle continues, a smoker adapts to these higher levels, reinforcing the need to smoke. In this way, the actual capability of these same biochemicals to respond to increasing stress has been diminished. In other words, nicotine use wastes the body's reserve and capability to maintain health's balance and defend against disease.

Dr. Pommerleau's data give us another important clue about the maladaptive nature of smoking. Despite the consistent increase of biochemicals which cause pleasure and alertness, biochemicals which strengthen our immunity response—our ability to fight disease and heal when we become ill—are not enhanced by smoking. The other bad effects of nicotine have been well-documented elsewhere. Thus, we needn't belabor the harms which smoking can cause.

It is interesting to note, again, that the biochemistry of happiness is now often linked with the biochemistry of health. However, in the case of nicotine enhanced pleasure, the body's immune strength does not correspond with euphoria. The other harmful effects of smoking continue to progress toward dis-ease processes within the lungs and circulation. Smokers use nicotine to feel good, to induce para-sympathetic biochemistry, to remain relaxed and alert, to be prepared for life's difficulties, to cope with stress. Through this artificial, euphoric substance, Endorphins and other fellow-biochemicals unfortunately reinforce the maladaptive, harmful use of biochemistry in the body. Through smoking, adaptation to he stress of life is falsely induced by the flow of euphoric biochemicals. Yet, this flow does not correspond with immune strength, and a disease process begins to corrode the maintenance of health.

Through an ongoing balance of parasympathetic and sympathetic biochemicals, we adapt to the stimulus of life. We've reviewed that stimulus can take the form of the physical stress of exercise and temperature change. Eating is a similar physical stimulus response, as are external substances like alcohol and nicotine—two forms of artificial stimulus which mimic this natural balance.

Tapping the Emotional Brain

Emotional and mental stimulus also affects the parasympathetic/sympathetic balance toward our well-being. To understand this, remember back to our Chapter One analogy of a mountain lake. Our mountain lake was a reservoir of thoughts and feelings—energy received from the incoming stimulus of our five senses. This reservoir holds memory impressions from previous stimulus, as well as incoming sensory impressions from present experiences. Both combine to become emotional content—flowing in biochemical rivers from this reservoir to influence the body.

This reservoir is analogous to the brain's middle layer, known as the *limbic brain*. Research has established this layer as being associated with our emotions of reward or punishment, as well as a primary regulatory mechanism of health. Stimulus within this brain center creates our experiences of pleasure and pain.

As you already might guess, this emotional limbic brain is the subject of intense study regarding Endorphins. Also, this brain region is rich with a wealth of Endorphin receptor sites or keyholes.

A Delicate Balance

You'll recall from Chapter One that Dr. Huda Akil touched the brains of her laboratory rats with an electrical stimulus. The carefully chosen site for this stimulus is found within the limbic brain. Dr. Akil's experiment utilized electricity which connected with the limbic brain to produce decreased perceptions of pain in these rats.

Another study involving stimulus to the limbic brain shows how an animal will reward itself with a certain learned behavior. Again, scientists painlessly inserted electrodes into the limbic brain region of experimental rats. This apparatus was connected to wires which the animals could trigger. Upon completion of specific laboratory mazes, the rats received an electrical stimulus from the apparatus connected with their limbic brains. This behavior was quickly learned and repeated by the rats. In fact, the animals frequently chose to run the maze rather than taking nourishment, because the electrical stimulus produced a limbic response of pleasure.

Endorphins again? Indeed, Endorphins have been found to be involved throughout the middle-layer or limbic brain. From what we already know about Endorphin potency, it is easy to understand why these laboratory animals would prefer the biochemical pleasure produced by electrical stimulus of their limbic brains. A task, a learned behavior, an electrically stimulated pleasure, a choice to go again—and a limbic cycle is developed, in which Endorphins reinforce this learned behavior.

Remember, as in Chapter One, back to a time when you had a happy experience which triggered a memory that remains vitally alive to you, even now. The original event was a stimulus that received an extra biochemical, electrical boost in its power, to remain ever-fresh in your mind. As we already have learned, your experience was underlined, or given strength, by a potent stimulus and a corresponding balance of biochemistry within your brain at that time. It was linked into your memory by a state of euphoria and excitement which you recorded in your brain. Endorphins are now implicated as the biochemicals responsible for the euphoric reward that bonded your brain to a strong memory.

In turn, these powerful pleasure memories help determine the choices we make—how we run our own mazes each day, sometimes even without nourishment. The stronger our pleasure-based memories are, the more likely we are to repeat behaviors associated with these memories. If you were brought up in a loving family environment, for instance, your memory of that experience affects your emotional choices in matters pertaining to family.

A similar mechanism may be involved in the negative stimulus of an emotional pain and a corresponding avoidance behavior. Consider a bad memory. This is one in which both fear and anxiety probably were present within your awareness. Again— this time because of the unpleasantness involved— stress-induced Endorphins may well have bonded your memory to that event. Several studies about fear-motivation and fear-behavior have conclusively linked Endorphins with the learning of what is called *avoidance response.*

A Delicate Balance

Again, using early childhood as an example, you may have had a consistent negative interaction with one or both of your parents. If so, your impressions of these memories can have a negative effect upon your emotional relationships. When we have an experience, which we do not want to have again, Endorphins—through their stress-induced biochemical reinforcement—help to create this avoidance response, assisting us to learn what we should avoid.

From this ongoing biochemistry of learning and memory, our brains process information to define both what we enjoy and what we would rather avoid. As our internal emotions are colored by our ongoing experiences, and vice versa, we make conscious and unconscious choices based upon continuous stimulus to and from the emotional limbic brain.

We know that Endorphins are involved in our sensations of pleasure, and perceptions of pain. Endorphins help us to adapt to stress. Adapting to the flow of life, we record past experiences, add new ones. Our behavior and choices reflect this emotional biochemistry, and we feel ourselves reinforced by (or avoiding) family, possessions, and even ideas and causes.

Through these adaptations, personality problems can emerge. The more we learn about Endorphins, and their addictive ability, the more we know that our adaptations can encourage us to develop personality imbalances in response to stress.

❊ ❊ ❊

The Ebb and Flow of Depression

For instance, as we have mentioned, Endorphins have been implicated in one of the most common personality imbalances, the condition called *depression*. Indeed depression is a disease of widespread proportions. Deep within this condition, there are both limitation and frustration over the limitation. It is as though the depressed person easily sinks further, getting worse and harder to help.

You may have known depressed people or may have experienced this feeling for yourself. While depressed, your being would seem to have diminished, no longer supplied with fresh inflow. Overcome by a limitation in flow, your enthusiasm and vitality would seem to have vanished. Even as you feel depleted, you might also feel irritable, or even hostile. From this condition, you would lapse into a feeling of standing still, waiting for the flow of life to happen to you once again.

It has long been known by the scientific community that mental illness, such as depression, is somehow an imbalance in the flow of the brain's biochemicals. To that end, many therapies have been devised to treat this imbalance by prescribing medications. These drugs have been developed and used in an attempt to change chemical imbalances within the brain. Unfortunately, many of these drugs have undesirable side effects. In some instances, they mimic missing biochemicals but do not yet completely simulate the biochemical balance experienced by a mentally well person.

The design of drugs for the treatment of mental illness is still in its infancy. Accordingly, mental health researchers have been quick to study Endorphins and their corresponding euphoria. But, although countless research hours have been spent and hundreds of articles written, easy answers have not been uncovered. From the data about Endorphins and depression, a complex puzzle about the nature of biochemical flow begins to emerge.

We can recognize the difference between a person who is depressed and someone who is enthusiastic. Energy and vitality radiate from a positive, enthusiastic person. Both qualities are notably absent in a pessimistic, depressed person. Following this concept, we would be inclined to ask—wouldn't depression seem to be characterized by a *lack* of Endorphins—where the flow of happiness and vitality would seem to be at at low ebb?

We might be tempted to think that because Endorphins relieve pain and create pleasure, the more Endorphins we have the better we feel. Surprisingly, however, many Endorphin researchers feel that depression can be caused by too many Endorphins.

Dr. S. Craig Risch and his colleagues have written a research review that cites many studies which show that depression is somehow linked with *increased* Endorphin levels. Their review underlines our previous explorations that high levels of Endorphins can be connected with an over-response of relaxation biochemicals. You'll recall our imagery of the picnic nap. After lying still for too long, you imagined feeling lethargic, numb to sensation, with a depressed sense of being alive. From this imagery, you sensed too much relaxation and rest. Parasympathetic biochemicals, possibly including Endorphins, over-predominate, too far out of balance.

However, other scientists have uncovered clues supporting our other observation that depression could be linked with low Endorphin levels. Researchers interested in reproductive cycles have noted a common malady following childbirth, called *post-partum depression.* Countless women have experienced this to some degree. They liken this sense of depression to a withdrawal from a bliss-inducing drug. They feel chronically irritable, close to tears, withdrawn, overwhelmed, and unmotivated by this new life in their lives.

As reviewed for the journal *Medical Hypotheses,* two Endorphin researchers, Dr. Uriel Halbreich and Dr. Jean Endicott, consider that post-partum depression would seem to be a true withdrawal from a previous high tide of euphoric Endorphins. During pregnancy, Endorphin levels rise significantly. This finding correlates with consistent reports that some women feel better when they are pregnant. Many have even noticed relief from chronic headaches during this nine-month cycle. Often, pregnancy is considered to be one of the happiest, most blissful times in a woman's life. From these reports, it is not unexpected that such happiness-biochemicals as Endorphins would increase during this time.

Pregnancy's increasing weight, drain of nourishment, and climax of painful labor are all major stressors upon the females of our species. Endorphins, increasing during pregnancy to be at their highest levels for the time of labor, would be a biochemical reward and reinforcement mechanism. The pain-killing effect of Endorphins assists the pregnant mother and encourages her to repeat the experience of motherhood.

At the end of pregnancy, the mother has just experienced nine months of increasing biochemical bliss. She has enjoyed the biochemical balance she has needed to survive a painful and, perhaps arduous, labor. As birth begins a new cycle of life, a biochemical change also occurs. The mother's post-partum depression, a possible withdrawal from high Endorphin levels, may well be similar to withdrawal from other addictions. Post-partum depression appears to be a biochemical-waiting for the return of fresh input—the flow of euphoria to reinforce and reward a continued commitment to life.

Further, as you'll recall from earlier material in Chapter Two, researchers at the University of Wisconsin are using the stress of exercise to improve the mood of those suffering from depression. From what we already know about parasympathetic/sympathetic responses in the body, this activation would be understandable. In an ongoing manner, one response balances the other—when parasympathetic biochemicals over-predominate, a stimulus is needed to initiate the opposite sympathetic flow. As the exercise study showed, a depressed person who is now running would feel a new sympathetic stimulus—a new flow of biochemical vitality.

Stimulus Again!

This stimulus toward balance might well be the beginning of a solution to our Endorphin puzzle about depression. On the one hand, depression would seem to be at a low ebb of euphoric biochemicals—on the other, high Endorphin levels also have been discovered in cases of depression.

These same high Endorphin levels have been associated with boredom, lethargy, and lack of motivation, the over-dominance of parasympathetic responses. Might these cases represent a lack of flow at a high level of biochemicals—like a lake that has a high water level but lacks a fresh stream of water to keep its contents free of stagnation?

This example from nature is a key to our understanding of Endorphins and depression. A stagnant lake lacks either the fresh input from a stream above its shores, or the ongoing outflow of a stream draining below. Parasympathetic stagnation, which seems to reinforce addiction to depression, may not lack the input of fresh stimulus, but may lack an outlet for expression of that same stimulus.

The other kind of depression, represented by withdrawal following pregnancy, might simply be a low ebb of Endorphins, where fresh input is needed. In either case, the recycling flow of stimulus could lead us to a solution for depression. Through incoming stimulus and its expression, both the stagnation and the low flow of depression could give way to a new biochemical impetus.

Pediatric researchers have uncovered another clue about biochemical depression and stimulus. As Endorphin levels have risen within the pregnant mother, so too do these biochemicals affect the fetal child. Within the mother's womb, a fetal child sleeps heavily, receiving oxygen supply from an umbilical link with the maternal bloodstream. A baby's first full breath is known to be taken after birth, when safe, oxygen-filled air is present to inflate the lungs.

Why wouldn't this fetal child inadvertently breathe deeply before birth? High Endorphin levels are now known to slow or *depress* respiration. From this knowledge, speculation is developing that pregnancy's increased Endorphin response is the reason why fetal children only breathe with shallow respirations, and thus avoid contaminating their lungs from their mothers' liquid-filled wombs.

A child is born, having spent nine months without breathing with its own developing lungs. Now, this one must breathe deeply to survive. Little, premature lungs are one of the risks a new baby faces, and many children are premature, or perhaps their lungs have developed slowly and are yet too immature for these babies to breathe deeply and well. Such a child's respiration is thus depressed, causing concern for his survival. (Remember that hearty crying is a good sign of strong, healthy lungs.)

High Endorphin levels, carried over from before birth, depress respiration and may keep some infants too deeply asleep, as though they were yet nourished from within the womb. Speculation about these continuing high Endorphin levels in infancy has led to evidence which links crib death to a corresponding ceasing of respiration. When these cases are discovered and recognized before death, stimulus may be used to awaken the infant and encourage deeper breathing.

Again, high Endorphin levels are correlated with parasympathetic over-predomination, drowsy, lethargic, needing the fresh flow of stimulus.

Piecing the Puzzle Together

We are engaged in learning how Endorphins flow to maintain health. In fascinating glimpses of new research now being reported, we have learned that Endorphins seem to help us respond to stress in adaptive ways. They reinforce our choices for reproduction. They are involved in appetite, and with nourishment as a reward. They give us parasympathetic ease. But, although it would be tempting to consider that high levels of Endorphins are always desirable, both high and low levels can represent undesirable imbalances.

An Endorphin insufficiency might be a biochemical source for depression—or, a high Endorphin level might become the stagnant pool in which lethargic depression begins. Put simply, lethargic, overly nourished people may have too many Endorphins, while anxious, undernourished people might feel Endorphin depletion. These are two extreme examples of a continuum that many people experience throughout their lives.

Biochemicals called Endorphins reinforce the wise or unwise choices that each of us makes. We have learned that a pleasure instinct hidden deep within the layers of the brain reinforces our learning, memories, and choices. If we choose to abuse alcohol, nicotine, and other harmful drugs, a complex biochemical chain of events in the body is created which may be a substitute for an imbalance of Endorphins.

Life continues on, changes flow from high to low ebb, to flow again and yet again. An ongoing stream of Endorphins continues—powerful, euphoric—designed to help us adapt to an ever-changing world. From these ideas, we can begin to piece the Endorphin puzzle together. In the next chapter we will explore further the biochemical reaction to stress, and how Endorphins may be utilized to help overcome our maladaptive responses to a stressful life.

❈ ❈ ❈

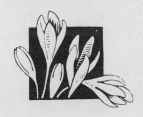

HOW-TO EXPLORATIONS TO TRY

—Remembering that extreme heat and cold can trigger Endorphins, use an ice pack or heating pad as home remedies for minor aches and pains. Often, these simple treatments are not given the respect they deserve, because, until now, the Endorphin relief of pain has not been understood. Be sure to follow your doctor's advice for appropriate applications.

—Recent findings have shown that increased exercise is an essential ingredient of a permanent weight-loss program. Exercise stimulates the sympathetic mode, increasing your biochemical metabolism. As you exercise, take note of that natural "high" Endorphins can give you. Use these pleasurable impressions to help reinforce your weight-loss program through consistent, increasing exercise.

—When you are tempted to use drugs because of peer pressure at school, or in your social circle, remember what you've learned about your natural Endorphin "high." You don't need drugs. You have your own natural biochemicals that are several hundred times more powerful than even morphine. Remember that you have Endorphins—appreciate them. Focus on triggering a natural "high" through new stimulus, exercise, activities, hobbies, and friends—new ways of experiencing life.

—If you smoke and wish to quit, take some time to think about why you smoke. Does it make you feel simultaneously relaxed and mentally alert? Ask yourself why you need these sensations—do you feel overly tense or mentally inadequate without the use of cigarettes? Write these impressions in a journal. Remember that your own natural biochemistry can flow without the stimulus of nicotine to help you feel comfortable and mentally sharp. Experiment with the stimulus of new activities and endeavors as you cut down or quit smoking. Take note of the activities that are most effective in helping you quit.

—Do you use alcohol to cope with the stress in your life? Remember that alcohol is a substitute way of inducing ease. Ask yourself what feelings you derive from drinking. Does alcohol help you feel un-inhibited, more acceptable—even loved? Does alcohol help you forget the troubles you perceive? How can you provide yourself the stimulus you need—without using an external substance? Keep a diary of your impressions.

—When you find yourself depressed, try to determine if your feeling stems from an overload of stimulus, (too many Endorphins) or a lack of stimulus (too few). Both problems represent the need for stimulating the opposite, sympathetic response. Remember that the stagnation or overload of too many Endorphins may require that you take action in some way to release the flow. One way is to find a new activity that will help you cope with the stimulus-overload you may be experiencing. In other instances, this stimulus-overload may represent thoughts and feelings which just need physical expression. In other instances, this stimulus-overload may represent thoughts and feelings which just need physical expression. In other instances, this stimulus-overload may represent thoughts and feelings which just need physical exprerssion. Be creative, develop constructive outlets for this pent-up stimulus.

On the other hand, the condition of too few Endorphins requires the flow of fresh stimulus, even though stimulus seems the last thing you want when you're depressed. Exercise is already a proven therapy. If you can't or won't exercise, *do* something—anything! Try something new and slightly challenging—a hobby, or volunteer work that encourages interaction with life. Read a new book on your favorite topic, or begin a new interest that you can then read more about. Working with animals is also therapeutic.

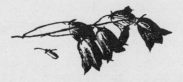

..we have learned that the body possesses a complex machinery of checks and balances. These are remarkably effective in adjusting ourselves to virtually anything that can happen to us in life. But often this machinery does not work perfectly: sometimes our responses are too weak, so that they do not offer adequate protection; at other times they are too strong, so that we actually hurt ourselves by our own excessive reactions to stress.

—Hans Selye, M.D.

— Three —

Following The
Endorphin Stream

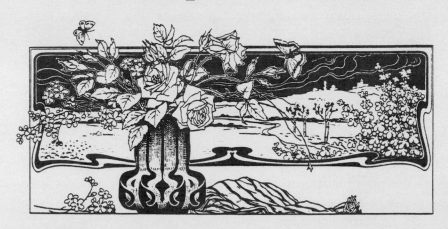

*W*inter, like all the seasons before, has come and is now departing. Slowly, the river thaws and begins to rise. Return now to the canyon of our imagery. The mountains ascending beside you have melting snow upon them. The desert at your feet lies waiting, thirsty as before. Although the place is the same and the boulders haven't moved, your vantage point is different. Gone is the stillness of autumn. Now, icy water overflows the rock where you once rested on a warm, summer day. Soon begins the surge of spring, and with it, change and growth.

Come close now to a ledge among the boulders where a swelling waterfall bursts down to the rocks below. Finding a place to stand close to the edge of the torrent, you even can taste and smell the spray upon your face. A rainbow from the sun shoots through the water. All you can hear is the din of the rising flood. A wind rushes through the canyon, brisk upon your face. Your senses join together to bring you the thrill of life's adventure.

Thus energized, your heart begins to beat faster; you can hear it pounding. You are stimulated by your own sense of springtime. Your body might tingle with expectation. Inspired to begin again, you feel a swell of desire for something new. Or you might perceive your old life in a new way. Your river of biochemicals runs differently now, dominated by a sense of stimulus. Because of this, you feel wonderfully alive, ready for almost anything—expectant.

Within this imagery, you have returned in Chapter Three to the same setting you envisioned in Chapter Two—the same rocks, the same background, maybe even the same recycled drops of water. Yet, your new perception of the feel of the place has initiated an entirely different biochemical response. This too is a stimulus-stress reaction, only now, invigorating. As we know, it is called the sympathetic or "fight or flight" response. From this bio-electrical stimulus, your senses are sharpened, even keen. Excited, you are ready to live and survive, with a rapid impulse for action. You are prepared to dare life head-on or to take quick action to flee. Of course, this is only an imagery, an exercise in perception. Your capacity to envision, using all of your five senses simultaneously, has kindled you with a feeling of excitement, challenge, or perhaps, even fear.

The biochemistry of the sympathetic nervous system has been represented by your vision. You probably noticed, right away, that this feeling is an exact opposite of the parasympathetic response you imagined that you had experienced in the last chapter. Your brain's government is designed to respond in these two opposite ways, prepared to adapt to life's requirements. Within and between these two responses, sympathetic and parasympathetic, lies a great pendulum swing of emotion and corresponding bodily reactions.

Discovering Eustress

Within the sympathetic condition of this swing, a sense of stress rises like a thawing stream. But, this stress does not yet seem overwhelming. It feels good, thrilling. Instead of feeling burned out or drowned by the rising tide of life, you might feel awakened, enlivened, ready for the swim.

In his study of stress concepts, Dr. Hans Selye has noticed this interesting difference in our perceptions of life's stress. His book *Stress Without Distress* explains his observations. Dr. Selye makes the distinction between two kinds of stress.

He noted that we tend to consider the concept of stress as some sort of ominous threat. We might perceive that stress is really generalized as life's crises. It might be those happenings that call up frustration, fear, and anger from within us; the happenings to which we feel powerless to respond constructively. This is the first kind of stress which Dr. Selye calls *distress*. It is a sense of being overburdened by events and closed in by unwelcome expectations thrust upon us. Today, as stress is a well-known commodity, it is blamed for all sorts of maladies, from ulcers to migraines, from heart disease to arthritis. Indeed, the distress side of stress might well be a predisposing factor to ill health.

Remembering back to Chapters One and Two, we recall that, as stress happens to us, a corresponding, rising tide of biochemical responses flows to help us cope. This is the cycle of adaptation to life. As we discussed at length, Endorphins are involved in our capacity to adapt. When we encounter a fight during this adaptation cycle, we might become wounded by events. But, powerful, pain-killing Endorphins often rise to help us meet these circumstances, and the possible pain is simply absent from our senses. If we choose to flee, we are stimulated to run hard; Endorphins are involved in the biochemical stamina required to do so, giving us a "high" or second wind to push harder and longer.

Within this adaptation, Endorphins may well help us to endure hardships, like the example of climate extremes studied in Canada. Endorphins are involved in the strengthening of immunity against the stressful onslaught of disease or injury. Also, Endorphins rise to help us to prepare psychologically, emotionally, and mentally for a perceived coming event where we anticipate a sense of stress. In one study reviewed at the Max-Planck Institute in West Germany, a significant rise in Endorphin blood levels was noted in students who felt stress from upcoming important examinations.

These Endorphin findings give us a clue about the second kind of stress which Selye identified. This is the stress that would make us feel euphoric, expectant, even thrilled about life. Even before Endorphins were discovered and identified, Dr. Selye noticed this important correlation between euphoria and stress. Thus, he termed his observation *eustress*.

What do we know about Endorphins that we can connect with eustress? Through the powerful biochemical capacity of Endorphins, stress is transformed into a rewarding experience, and is thus perceived as eustress. The tide of life's challenge rises, and we can rise with it, feeling stimulation, excitement, and pleasure, as if flowing over rocks and cresting up, rafting the Endorphin river with the exhilaration of shooting white-water rapids.

As we find ourselves successfully adapting within the cycle of life's stress, eustress reinforces itself. We begin to seek out challenge, to call it to us. We enjoy the stimulus, missing it when a crisis is over. Thus, a sense of addiction to life begins. We are glad to be alive, feeling pleasure in waking, getting up, walking, running to interact. We say, "Just let life come, we are prepared."

As we succeed, we become biochemically bonded by a euphoria that reinforces our sense of life. Somehow, Endorphins play a major role in this addiction. Our perception about ourselves and life's eustress encourages behavior which responds with an adaptation capacity to rise, grow, and learn.

Many of us appreciate eustress each day. We work and play hard, enjoying the action. A good stream of brain biochemicals flows to reinforce our motivation to do, and our rewarded experience reinforces our motivation to go again. With each passing stressor successfully challenged, our capacity to adapt is reinforced to perceive the stress as eustress. The flow continues. People who enjoy high achievement and hard work have learned to use this biochemical cascade of eustress to feel good.

But, careful now, for the flow is accelerating. It is as though a warming trend has melted all the snow banks at once. No longer can we easily imagine standing beside the cascade to enjoy its spray upon our faces.

Envision a river rushing where you stood, overflowing its banks. What once seemed a din of noise is now a thunderclap resounding in your ears. Flashflood conditions prevail and threaten. The current thrashing river could carry you away as though you were a pebble.

Workaholism and Endorphins

The sympathetic response of biochemistry can become a flash-flood too. The moderate dose of stress might no longer be enough to feel good and motivated. Endorphins and addiction? The concept returns to plague us again. Initially, a small dose of eustress is taken. Simple enough at first, a challenging workday is well met. But now this level of stress becomes a baseline for feeling good. A greater fix is needed, a new project added, the challenge greater, the eustress more rewarding. Perhaps this lasts awhile, perhaps it does not. More eustress, and more! No more weekends relaxing. Keep business as usual, seven days a week.

Soon, one forgets when to stop, the eustress feels so good. The pain of overwork is not experienced. Endorphins, powerful pain-killers, may mask the warning symptoms. As in the further, harder push of marathon training, the "second wind" or "high" becomes a third and yet a fourth—miles and weeks of stress down the line. This is a syndrome already established in highly stressed people who are at risk for heart disease. Chest pain? Not much to speak of, hardly noticed it. Eustress masks the symptoms of impending distress and beginning disease processes.

Pushing harder and longer, the workaholic tests stress limits even as the heroin addict seeks higher and more frequent doses. Our bodies are designed with intrinsic biochemicals to reinforce the behavior that makes us feel good, even when this action goes too long and too far to stay healthy.

Returning to Dr. Selye's observations, he has noticed that our capacity to adapt to stress can vary. Every time we adapt to stress, our capability to adapt to additional stress is reduced. This stress cycle ends at some point of exhaustion. The length of this adaptation phase and its endurance is an individual response. A depressed person, who becomes distressed easily, is lethargic, depleted of internal biochemicals that reinforce resilient vitality. Because of this depletion, depression may block adaptation to a simple stressor, even for a day.

But, in an opposite example, the enthusiastic workaholic might endure even beyond the point of distress. Thus, a great stressor might not even be noticed, and a subsequent disease process could gain an unfortunate foothold. You will notice that both responses to stress are extreme.

Is "workaholism" a true addiction, rewarded and reinforced by the body's own biochemicals rather than external substances?

We have discussed addiction frequently in earlier chapters. Several points seem important to review. The potential for addiction lies within each of us. Powerful, intrinsic biochemicals reward our bonding, learning, and behavior. The addictive abuse of substances is an unfortunate example of an external response to this internal design.

Remember from earlier chapters that, within the nature of addiction, there is a significant adaptive cycle. With drug addiction, the tolerance/dependence cycle is externally induced, obvious to the bystander and of great concern. But, with workaholism, the internal addiction seems more subtle, for now the addictive dose comes from powerful internal biochemicals induced by learned behavior.

Two Endorphin researchers at the University of California, Irvine, Larry Stein and James D. Belluzzi, have correlated learned behavior with reward and the addictive potential of Endorphins. To design this experiment, Stein and Belluzzi used Enkephalins, a special group of brain biochemicals within the Endorphin family. Using laboratory rats and levers which the animals could press spontaneously, the researchers gave dosages of synthetic Enkephalin when the levers were pressed. No prior learning about this lever-press behavior had been established in these rats. The experiment developed substantial evidence that the animals became addicted to the lever-press behavior through the pleasure created by the Enkephalin doses.

Next, through electrodes placed where Enkephalins are known to originate, the lever-press behavior electrically stimulated an internal Enkephalin response. A similar addictive cycle was documented, evidence that, in both cases, Enkephalins were the biochemical reinforcers of behavior that became addictive.

We will return to the work of Stein and Belluzzi in later concepts. For now, their Enkephalin-induced behavioral addiction studies give us further clues. Endorphins have a very real potential to bond us to behavior, learned and reinforced by euphoria.

Reinforcing Pleasure

A child grows, responding to his environment. During this interaction, bonding and learning take place. Throughout this ongoing process, the child is biochemically reinforced to do what feels good and avoid what feels bad. Different kinds of behavior become habits and habits become habit-forming. These cycles can reinforce healthy behavior, bringing us much fulfillment and happiness.

But, there is no guarantee that what we enjoy feeling, thinking, and doing will necessarily be good for ourselves and our society. From this further clarification of reinforcement through euphoric biochemistry, deviant behavior, such as criminal acts, is better understood. Criminals seem compelled, in many cases, to commit dire crimes. It is as though they experience compulsion from within, addicted to these deviant kinds of behavior. Thus, Endorphins and other similar brain biochemicals could run amok, reinforcing the distressing diseases of society.

Of less concern to society but certainly a problem for each of us are those compulsive feelings, thoughts, and kinds of behavior we carry with us. We may often feel stuck with habitual ways of doing and being. Perhaps we feel compelled to be excessively organized (or disorganized). We say, "I have to have it just so" or "I never do it that way." Having learned already about biochemical reinforcement, we could say that we are addicted to these compulsions.

The tolerance/dependence cycle, ever-active, continues on, adding new layers of thoughts, feelings, and behavior. This often unconscious process, developing from responses to stress in the past, reinforces compulsions that become inflexible and unresponsive to present and future stress. From this trend, a rigid, unadaptable personality and lifestyle can develop.

Life continues on, change continues to change

again, requiring adaptation and growth of all that lives. As Dr. Selye has documented, our biochemical adaptation capacity is intrinsically designed to respond to the stress of change. Eustress may be defined as a euphoric response to the challenge of change. Distress may simply be the same stressor, perceived as overwhelming, beyond our control, or threatening to that part of ourselves which has been biochemically adapted or reinforced to inflexibly resist change.

From this model, eustress and distress are simply definitions or value judgments about the stress of life. All of us make these judgments every day in big and little ways. Our perceptions of stress mold our life's quality to a great degree. For example, most of us would consider falling thirty feet to be a great distressor. But the trapeze artist would consider that same experience to be just one small and pleasurable moment of eustress in a day's work. The difference lies in learned behavior, corresponding belief about one's capacities, and a constructive attitude to life, itself.

As the living process continues on, beliefs and attitudes successfully or unsuccessfully reinforce our doing and being. Eustress and distress, both biochemical occurrences, are beliefs or perceptions about our own responses to life's challenge. To help us make the distinction between eustress and distress, let's look further at how the brain has been designed with a distress-producing conflict deep within it.

✽ ✽ ✽

The Instinctual Brain

We could point to many external reasons why we might feel stress to a point of distress. We live in a stressful age or time in history. The sense of pending concern, challenge, or doom touches us at various levels of our experience. We feel stressed by world conditions. We are made more aware of these stress-producing causes through television's incessant and unrelenting international and local coverage of troubling events. We feel stress from our community troubles and family situations. No one of us seems to lead a simple life anymore. There is a complexity and, sometimes, even chaos about the environment around us, both in the world at large and within the circle of our closest relationships.

Despite these external stressors, the greatest challenge that we each individually realize is that sense of distress found within ourselves. Scientists now are beginning to understand how the brain, itself, may be the reason why we experience distress. Hidden deep within the brain, below and often in conflict with the middle, emotional/limbic layer we've learned about in Chapter Two, lies the *brainstem*, which maintains our physiological survival, and profoundly affects our instinctual self-preservation.

The brainstem is the body's life-preserver, regulating breathing and heartbeat, thus making sure that adequate oxygen is supplied throughout the brain and body. The brainstem is so essential to life that, when a stroke or other injury occurs within its borders, chances for survival are marginal and life-support mechanisms, such as respirators, must be used to maintain vital functions. When someone survives this interruption of brainstem process, a comatose, "vegetable," existence occurs. This kind of coma results because of blockage in brainstem communication and a corresponding lack of information to the higher layers of the brain responsible for consciousness.

Until recently, this deepest layer of brain was not considered to carry any kind of consciousness. It was known simply to regulate life-sustaining function. But now, according to Dr. Paul MacLean, the director of brain evolution and behavior at the National Institute of Mental Health in Bethesda, Maryland, the brainstem is considered to be the physical center for unconscious kinds of behavior and responses.

According to Dr. MacLean's theory, this deepest of brain layers is a relic of an instinctual form of life, still active within us. Dr. MacLean has called this structure the *reptilian brain*, named for its primitive origin and function.

There is now evidence that this deep layer of brain is responsible for the kinds of subconscious behavior which surprise us with the intense self-preserving mechanisms of hostility or territorial possessiveness and control. Dr. MacLean's observations include over twenty identifiable kinds of behavior which link our survival with the survival of our earliest ancestors. These include establishing territory, foraging, storing, growling, greeting, and forming groups, to name a few. According to Dr. MacLean's theory, when we find ourselves responding with these instinctive approaches to life, our reptilian brainstem—with its eons of conditioning—is functioning from an aggressive or defensive process that it once needed to survive.

We still experience the biochemical imperatives of our reptilian brain, which can emerge to give us a sense of distress, conflict, or challenge. We seek to placate this distress by focusing outside of ourselves, impelled to exert external power or control over our physical environment—the working world, finances, co-workers, and even our families. Although a sense of self-worth is necessary, this primitive sense of power may become an obsession, addictive like workaholism, stress-producing and potentially destructive.

Perhaps, more subtly, we may feel impelled to take territorial power over our own subconscious sense of ourselves. Thus, we can often feel hounded, perceiving that we must somehow run from, or to, something. But this is a vague notion, not easily explained nor analyzed. This "running" takes many forms, such as the compulsion to conform to a rigid diet, to run farther, work faster, or to force our lifestyles into a certain pattern.

Our instinct to control, filters into our sense of identity; we are strict with ourselves, punishing ourselves with guilt when we haven't measured up to a standard we have set for ourselves, our possessions, behavior, thoughts, and emotions. Or, we might feel a loss of control over any or all of these, fearful that we will never "make the grade." Again, this is the "grade" we have subconsciously set in order to control ourselves. And, when we fail, or believe that we do, that sense of failure or loss of territorial identity reinforces a sense of distress.

Distress is also present when we feel lack or failure emotionally, mentally, or even spiritually. We say, "I'm a terrible person for having that bad thought or hateful feeling." or, "I failed the standard again." And worse, we believe ourselves. We find ourselves compelled to be in that distressful frame of mind, where our physiology biochemically responds to reinforce negative feelings about "failure." Through this chain of negative perceptions, a sense of uncontrolled stress begins.

As this vicious cycle continues, our compulsions build to make us want to run, to withdraw in fear, or lash out to fight in anger. It is through this automatic mechanism that we feel that sense of "fight or flight" within our bodies. Through this physiological, yet often unconscious, process, all of our choices—indeed, our whole lives—can be oriented around these perceived priorities of failure, the subconscious loss of our sense of control over ourselves and our environment.

The Conflicting Brains

Dr. MacLean's observations show us that the brain is really comprised of three brains, each one with its own priorities, each with its own corresponding biochemistry. Each has its own individual effect upon our perceptions, our sense of eustress or distress. Each directly affects our physiology with automatic responses. The outermost brain layer is called the *cortex*—the one distinguishing us as human beings. It thinks, plans, analyzes, and gives us, we hope, a rational view of our world. Through the cortex, we are conscious of our world, consider its possibilities, and review its happenings.

But, it is from deeper layers of the brain that we obtain a sense of ourselves in relationship to the world. The middle, emotional/limbic layer is that potent place where feelings and sensations, impressions of the world's effect upon us, are recorded. As was previously stated, many potent brain biochemicals have their origins in this region, reinforcing our feelings and sensations with a powerful sense of euphoria or a distressing sense of lack or longing. Within this important region of emotional biochemistry, we bond to our loves and avoid or reject our hates, thus setting in motion a corresponding physiological response to our limbic priorities.

Hidden deep within our heads, biochemicals process feeling states which continue to flow beyond conscious, cortical awareness. The stress-and-pain research pharmacologist, whom we met in Chapter Two, Dr. Agu Pert, reminds us that it is within the limbic region that the emotional component of distress and pain is perceived. These same distress biochemicals can also erupt into disease processes.

The cortex, which maintains our everyday consciousness, can be unaware of the biochemical priorities of the emotional/limbic brain. And so, feelings and sensations can remain unconscious; or they somehow don't seem rational or logical to the cortical thinking process. Especially if we have been reinforced to feel good about our thinking capacities, we can become dominated by our intellect. Our feelings and sensations may even seem worrisome, or a bother, at best. Bad feelings and sensations, those we have learned to avoid, may be downright threatening to the thinking cortex. Thus a cortical "lid" is placed upon limbic processes so we don't have to think about or experience feelings and sensations. But the emotional/limbic brain continues on, receiving sensory input and reinforcing a feeling mode which always affects the body and its health, even when we are consciously unaware of this process.

As described earlier in detail, even deeper and often threatening to both feelings and thoughts, the instinctual reptilian brainstem carries on its own life. Drives for self-preservation, possession, and territory maintain their own subconscious biochemical priorities. This instinctive layer within each of us takes its own responsibility for the regulation of that "beast of burden" which is the physical body. If this beast's self-preservation is threatened, a distress perception begins a physiological response. From this theory, we can better understand why our bodies seem to betray us. The heart pounds when we perceive a threat, even if it's just a threat to the ego.

❊ ❊ ❊

Symptoms and Diseases
of Conflict

Tension can build within these feelings of conflict and their biochemical priorities. And, if this tension continues in a chronic pattern, our physiological distress responses eventually turn the body against itself. Many of us are plagued with muscle-tension symptoms as we perceive stress rising about us or feel it welling up within us. We know that stress triggers Endorphins that are intended to help us adapt to life's challenges. But, this ongoing adaptation to conflict can take a chronic toll for which the body eventually must pay. You'll recall Dr. Selye's stress theory—there is, within each of us, a level of distress triggering the end of our own individual stress adaptation limit.

Because Endorphins often have been linked with ease and the euphoric mood, scientists have been quick to consider tension and stress diseases as indications for loss of adaptation and for possible Endorphin depletion, or stagnation of Endorphin flow.

Researchers in Italy have focused upon the well-known migraine headache in this regard. In a paper published in *Advances in Neurology*, Dr. A. Agnoli and his colleagues note that a heroin-withdrawal headache is described as similar to a migraine. This clue would indicate that migraine headache might be some sort of Endorphin limitation. Although these experiments confirm other studies showing that the migraine process is complex beyond a simple Endorphin depletion, Dr. Agnoli and his colleagues were able to reverse the pain of a migraine headache with the use of synthetic Enkephalin (a member of the Endorphin family).

In another, related, article, a team of Endorphin researchers working together from Milan and Florence noted naturally occurring, high Endorphin levels when the migraine crisis ends and freedom from pain returns.

Ulcers are another chronic problem attributed to tension and a distress response to stress. We already have learned about the important connection between Endorphins and the digestive system. High Endorphin levels are correlated with slow digestion, slow metabolism, and subsequent obesity. From these known high levels, we might consider that low levels of Endorphins could be correlated with gastric stress disorders like ulcers, Crohn's disease and ulcerative colitis. Explaining in an article for the journal *Gastroenterology*, Drs. R.F. Ambinder and Marvin Schuster see this link between Endorphin depletion and digestive irritability as a real possibility.

Again, considering heroin-withdrawal digestive symptoms, these physicians show that similar symptoms are commonly seen in irritable intestinal syndromes. Gastroenterologists often hear patients complain of major digestive symptoms, only to find from their studies that there is no disease process. These gastric and intestinal symptoms are termed *functional* rather than *pathological*. Drs. Ambinder and

Schuster point to Endorphin imbalances as the probable biochemical support for functional, yet distressing, digestive disorders.

From these beginning clues about Endorphin depletion and chronic disorders, it is not surprising to find that arthritis also would be on the research list. At a recent meeting of the Arthritis Foundation, Dr. Charles Denko described a correlation between Endorphin levels and several arthritic conditions. As noted in a 1981 issue of *Science News*, Dr. Denko and his colleagues have reported significantly low Endorphin levels in both blood and joint fluids of patients with rheumatoid arthritis, osteoarthritis, gout, and other rheumatic diseases. This low level was compared and standardized against the Endorphin levels of healthy people. Especially low Endorphin levels were discovered in some arthritic conditions with severe pain.

Dr. Denko goes on to explain that his findings about Endorphins show that high levels correlated with optimism, low levels with pessimism. Other arthritis researchers have noticed that a positive self-image improves the probability of improvement for arthritis patients. The negative view makes progress for the arthritis victim more difficult. Dr. Denko feels that Endorphins are important brain biochemicals to study for the future of arthritis treatment.

A Change in Perception

Through powerful biochemical priorities, there arise within us, motivations, desires, compulsions, challenges, and conflicts. We are so designed, biologically. We pace, we seek, we long after some external toy or pleasure. We seek outside ourselves for someone or something, an external happiness. Our five senses are designed to make this so.

As you'll recall from Chapter One, our five senses send information that is really electrical stimulus, acting as a communication signal to tell us about the compelling world around us. Through this biochemical, electrical process, we relate to our world. Experience thus begins and continues throughout a lifespan. The brain's environment, brain biochemistry in general, and Endorphins in particular, reinforce and even shape our external impressions. Through this ongoing process, we somehow choose what we love, what we love doing, and to whom or to what we bond. Our perceptions trick us into thinking and feeling that it is the external source or object of our love that makes us feel happy. But it is really the pleasure biochemically reinforced from within that gives a sense of fulfillment when we obtain what we seek after.

Have you ever found yourself feeling stale in a relationship or situation or possession you formerly have treasured? Where once you felt a thrill, an exhilaration, a bonding, a reinforcing, now you feel a lack, a loss of vitality. It is as though the essence of this external love has evaporated away. But what really represents this loss? A vague sense of longing, once fulfilled by one or all of these treasures, signals an adaptive biochemical response. Now this same longing wells up again, seeking after a new happiness.

In this way, we can see the tolerance/dependence cycle afflicting each of us, as well as the addict. But the change of feeling we notice reflects a change inside ourselves, not a change in the external environment, even though it seems so. The feeling-change is a shift in brain biochemistry, perhaps from a deep limbic or reptilian brain process.

No longer do we feel biochemically euphoric in response to that stimulus, where happiness seemed to have been. Developing a tolerance to that previous stimulus, we have changed, and with that change we seek again to grow toward new territory, new identity, and new meaning to life. If we do not follow after new impetus, a vague sense of staleness can grow instead, bonding us again, from an internal biochemical reinforcement, to lack of stimulus—to that rut our lifestyle begins to become.

Sometimes we bond to something or someone, becoming biochemically immersed in our sense of loving. Again, euphoric biochemistry reinforces our joy. We believe again, with a slip in perception, that this joy is external. We forget that happiness comes from within. We love our family, our friends, our careers, the environment in which we find ourselves. We know great joy reverberating in the loving. And miraculously, we also know health and a fine quality of life.

But then, as always, the seasons change. Life continues on. All at once, change happens to us. We lose a loved one; we're forced to retire or move. A fire burns our beloved home. A thief in the night steals our precious jewels. An economic wind blows investment away. The supposed external stimulus evaporates.

At this point, a biochemical state of distress can begin, increasing in proportion with each negative *psychological response* to stress. These stressors can build or accumulate to a point identified by Dr. Selye as the end of our adaptation capacity. When this point is approached, even through subconscious emotional or instinctual conflicts, our bodily responses are weakened and depleted. We slowly lose our strength of adaptability. And with that loss, we can also lose our strength of *immunity*—our capability to maintain health by defending against disease.

The Immunity Connection

During the earliest research about Endorphins, it was discovered that our responses to stress, the strength of our immunity, and the flow of Endorphins are interconnected. To learn about how Endorphins are linked to immunity, let's briefly recall our imagery in Chapter One. Our biochemical processes are like an ongoing river of microscopic events.

Again, picture the flow of hormones to be like a cascading waterfall. Its headwaters begin within the brain's hypothalamus, the body's master hormonal gland. This hormonal current flows into the *pituitary gland*, stimulating the production of many hormones which then run throughout the rest of the body via the bloodstream. From this ongoing process, hormones or biochemical messengers flow to affect our health. The hormonal messages of immunity are some of the most important of these ongoing communications throughout the body.

A hormone researcher happened upon the Endorphin/immunity clue while simultaneously finding a now-famous specific Endorphin. At the University of California, San Francisco, Dr. Choh Hao Li discovered the Endorphin called *Beta-Endorphin*. It is a small but powerful segment of a longer hormonal chain arising from the pituitary gland.

Dr. Li's discovery of Beta-Endorphin was exciting enough. But, within this discovery, Dr. Li hit upon a research jackpot. Here, within the longer hormone chain, Beta-Endorphin's next-door neighbor was discovered to be a hormone called *adrenocorticotrophic hormone*, or *ACTH*, for short. ACTH is a small and powerful hormonal chain of chemical keys which contributes greatly to our health by unlocking ongoing immunity signals throughout our bodies.

At once, researchers began to study this surprising health-maintenance clue. ACTH is an immune hormone which is triggered into action by stress. Now, researchers know that stress triggers the release of Beta-Endorphin, as well. Many studies about the connections between Endorphins, immunity, and stress have been made since that first discovery. As stress triggers the co-release of Beta-Endorphin with ACTH, we can understand why an increasing exercise program would help to keep us healthy by strengthening immunity. This could also be the reason why stopping an exercise program might increase susceptibility to colds and flu.

In a theory called *immune surveillance*, immunity is credited with more than an ability to fight infections like colds and flu. This theory claims, for example, that immunity normally has the strength to fight cancer before is becomes a disease. Potentially cancerous cells lie within each of us. Through immune surveillance, these tiny, malignant threats are checked by a strong immune defense. Thus, the out-of-control malignant growth that becomes a cancerous disease process is linked with an immune depression which fails to defend against the rising tide of malignancy.

In a book about immunity, *The Body is The Hero*, Dr. Ronald J. Glasser describes the immune surveillance theory. For supporting evidence, Dr. Glasser cites two specific age groups that are well known to have greater immune deficiencies. Often, advancing age weakens bodily systems, especially immunity, making older people more susceptible to illness. Young children can have immature, not fully developed, bodies, also more susceptible to disease. The very elderly and the very young are often unable to maintain the strength of immune surveillance, then becoming susceptible to cancer and other immune-depleted ailments.

Other evidence for immune surveillance suggests that organ-transplant patients, receiving immune-suppressive drugs for the sake of reducing a transplant rejection, have a statistically larger chance of also developing cancer. Likewise, it has been documented that when an immune-suppressant drug therapy was discontinued, a fast-growing malignancy stopped its advance and the patient gained a remission.

There are established cases of cancer patients who have gained remissions simultaneously while experiencing additional virulent infections. In these cases, it can well be speculated that a powerful infectious process might provide the stimulus which a previously unresponsive immunity would need to combat an underlying insidious malignancy. This kind of evidence leads to the proposal that vaccines which strengthen immunity may prove to be a realistic cancer treatment, and more research is needed.

Linking Emotions and Health

But might there be an emotional cause for immune depletion such that a few cancer cells could grow into an advanced disease process? This question was asked by Dr. R. W. Banthrop, an immunity researcher from New South Wales, Australia. His graphic study was detailed in a 1977 issue of a British medical journal, titled *Lancet*.

In 1976, a bridge in Australia collapsed. This was an especially unfortunate event because a train was crossing the bridge as it fell. Many train passengers were killed. Dr. Banthrop, who already had wondered about the connection of mind and emotions with biochemistry, used this tragedy to study his ideas. He went to the scene of the accident and sought permission to take blood samples of some of the survivors whose spouses had been killed. Those people who allowed their blood to be studied were then researched over the next six weeks. The bereaved wives and husbands, ranging in age from twenty-five to sixty-five, were compared with a "control" group of hospital employees who had not experienced this loss.

Dr. Banthrop and his colleagues found that the resulting comparison showed a significant depletion in the lymphocyte count of the bereaved subjects. The lymphocyte is a specific white cell within blood components known to be an important immunity line of defense against disease. A catastrophic event, especially as perceived by those who had lost their wives and husbands, had consistently initiated a beginning depression of the immune strength that maintains biochemical health.

Endorphins are connected with our subjective sense of loss and bereavement. (The euphoria of Endorphins is associated with caring, love, and bonding.) An overwhelming catastrophy, such as the one studied by Dr. Banthrop, should clearly have some effect on Endorphin levels, as well as on immune strength.

When we lose someone or something we love, we become depressed emotionally for a time. It would be tempting to think that this emotional depression can be directly correlated with a loss of

Endorphins. After all, when one is grieving, happiness and the feeling of joy about life seems far removed from present conditions. This depressive loss appears to be a depletion of euphoria, or low Endorphin levels.

However, based on what we've already learned, Endorphin levels can rise in response to stress. Indeed, a rising tide of Endorphins may well be the initial response to an overwhelming catastrophy such as the train wreck studied by Dr. Banthrop. (If you have experienced a major loss in your life, you might remember an initial response of numbness, or shock—a sense of unreality. This could be due, in part, to initially high Endorphin levels.)

But what happens next? Each of us responds to our losses in different ways, just as we respond to stress in different ways. This variation in response is the key to our question.

Two immunology researchers have considered our question in detail. Dr. Steven F. Maier, at the University of Colorado, in Boulder, and Dr. Mark Laudenslager, at the University of Denver, have written a review article called "Stress and Health: Exploring the Links" for a recent issue of *Psychology Today*.

Drs. Maier and Laudenslager explain that stress, or more specifically, distress, cannot be defined simply as a negative event, even the loss of a loved one, as studied by Dr. Banthrop. As we already have begun to explore, our responses to negative events become critical factors in our interactions with life's challenges. This response, or the *way* stress is perceived, may well be a key influence upon biochemical strength against disease.

A sense of control over the stressor has been identified as a potentially healthy response. At Duke University School of Medicine, Dr. Jay M. Weiss, a research psychologist, has studied animals in stressful situations. When animals are given control over unpleasant stimuli, they do not develop the physiological symptoms related to stress, such as ulcers and sleep disturbances.

A similar finding has recently been described by Dr. Kenneth Pelletier, a research physiologist from the University of California, San Francisco. While conditioning astronauts for the stressors of space, NASA developed a comparison study. Some astronauts were told that they would have no control over the events that would be simulated—that they simply would have to learn to respond to these stressors as best they could. Other astronauts were given a lever to activate when these same simulations became too stressful.

As we would expect, the group who could take lever-control over their simulation remained more relaxed during the tests. However, this lever was actually never connected into the mechanisms that affected the ongoing space simulations. The belief in the lever was the key factor in these relaxed stress responses.

A syndrome called *learned helplessness* has been identified as the opposite response to a sense of uncontrolled stress. Dr. Maier and Dr. Martin Seligman, a colleague from the University of Pennsylvania, have studied this syndrome. When animals are first conditioned to have no control over stress, they later have no ability to perceive an escape from stress when it becomes available. They remain passively helpless, unable to learn stress-avoidance behavior.

Further, data about immune strength have been collected from animals who have learned to be helpless. In one study, animals were unable to reject an implanted tumor (a predetermined sign of immune weakness) when they had previously been exposed to uncontrolled stressors. This finding would correlate with Dr. Banthrop's train wreck study about decreasing lymphocyte counts during a grieving period—when a bereaved person has no control over loss.

Dr. Maier has also studied the biochemical connections between Endorphins and learned helplessness. Animals who have been exposed to uncontrolled stress exhibit diminished pain sensitivity. The use of Endorphin drug antagonists later reversed this process, thus increasing pain. Interestingly, increased Endorphin levels have been implicated in the syndrome of learned helplessness.

Similar studies have used Endorphin antagonists to keep uncontrolled stressors from suppressing immune responses. The depressed immune response in uncontrolled stress has also been blocked by Endorphin antagonists. Further, lymphocytes are now known to possess Endorphin keyholes—yet another indication that these cells are involved in the communication between Endorphins and immunity.

This finding about lymphocytes, specialized white blood cells, takes us back to Dr. Banthrop's data following the train wreck. You'll recall that white blood cells decreased in the grieving individuals who were studied. If Endorphin levels did rise in response to the stress of the train wreck, as we can well suspect, this rise might have triggered a communication with the body's white blood cells, flooding their receptor sites with information that would eventually cause their decrease.

The clue to the maintenance of health during stressful periods still seems to be found in the variations of response to these stressors. At Harvard University Medical School, Dr. Steven Lock and his colleagues have developed a study about healthy people and their responses to stress. The subjects were given a questionnaire which indicated both the recent occurrence of stress and any emotional reactions to these events. Additionally, individual blood samples tested the immune strength of these subjects.

As measured in these samples, immune strength did not necessarily correlate with the frequency of major life-stressors. The key factor was emotional response.

Those who reported depression, anxiety, and many life-stressors also showed decreased immune strength. Those who did not report anxiety and depression, but also reported extensive life stresses, showed a high degree of immune strength.

This finding became even more significant when compared with those who reported that they were not stressed, anxious, or depressed. Immune strength was measured highest in those who reported a positive emotional reaction to extensive stress.

Clearly, our biochemical balance and the strength of our immunity are intimately linked with our deep emotional responses to life. Our biochemistry is influenced by our perception of stress and life's challenges. When we feel stuck in a negative response to stress, or incapable of dealing with our problems, how can we influence our biochemistry to a more positive flow?

The Imagery Connection

In their book *Getting Well Again*, two imagery researchers, Dr. Carl O. Simonton, and Stephanie Matthews-Simonton, explore our question. These researchers provide us with an example of how our brains function to release us from the distress states which can lead to disease.

Imagination is the product of biochemical brain processes. A memory of a past event or the planning of a future one—two common uses of the brain's imagery ability—are real biochemical events with real physiological effects.

The Simontons use this imagery concept in their treatment of cancer patients. They teach visualization and meditation techniques in an attempt to reprogram their client's emotional, biochemical processes. They encourage their clients to envision immune strength through symbolic and literal imageries of immune cells gaining force to become again a strong defense against disease. They urge their clients to reverse emotional hopelessness and unconscious loss with new imagery that strengthens biochemical happiness and reduces biochemical longing.

An exercise suggested by Dr. Neil Fiore, a psychologist who shared his findings at a University of California conference in San Francisco, incorporates this use of mental imagery. We can use Dr. Fiore's exercise which follows to clarify our own understanding of this process.

Imagine, now, a lemon tree that is filled with ripe lemons. Walk up to this tree and reach out to pick the best of the fruit that you can reach. Pluck the fruit from the tree, listen for the brush of leaves. Feel the lemon heavy in your hand. Notice the bright yellow peeling, which feels bumpy to your touch. Now, tear open the peeling and, smelling the sharp odor, find the juicy fruit awaiting your tasting.

Of course, the tree and fruit are only imagined experiences. However, the mind process initiates a host of biochemical brain responses which prepare your mouth for that lemon. This fountain of biochemistry brings an actual pucker response and saliva preparation for the tart lemon, whether it is imagined or not. Furthermore, your own previously acquired taste or dislike of the strong lemon flavor determines your response to it. This pre-determination results in a sense of enjoyment or distaste for this lemon imagery.

Were you really reaching for a real lemon on a real tree, or was this vivid experience only in your imagination? Well, of course it was imaginary—your conscious mind knows this—but—your brain's biochemical response did not differentiate and your mouth puckered up from the "sour taste" of the imaginary lemon. Nor was there a distinction made, by the brain's biochemistry, between the sensory awareness of a present happening and the sensory memory of a past experience with lemons. Your brain simply gave you the biochemical response you needed for that lemon taste. A biochemical communication, triggered by your mental imaging, delivered information to your salivary glands and tongue.

In a study that echoes the theme of our lemon imagery, it was discovered that imagery influences digestive processes. The envisioning of a steak dinner has the same effect upon increasing insulin secretion as does a serving of the real thing.

We can see, from our own exploration of Endorphin concepts, how therapeutic imagery could well have a profound influence upon our bodies. We know that positive emotions may be correlated with immune strength. We also know that this imagery is a biochemical mental activity affecting the brain's regulation of our bodies.

Sometimes, however, especially when we are ill, it's difficult to understand how our mental processes, concepts, or visions can influence our bodies. This intellectual exercise can seem far removed from our physical sense of distress, disease, or pain.

But, as we have discovered already, cortical thinking is not the only aspect of our complex psychology. The sum of psychological influences upon our ultimate health or disease is the sum of all the brain's priorities mixed together. Our psychology is composed of this bio-electrical bath of chemicals arising from all three of our brain layers—cortex, limbic, and reptilian. Although our eustress might easily be triggered through the mental stimulation of cortical activity, our sense of distress and pain often comes from deeper, hidden, and more subtle aspects of our psychological nature. Disease processes, which are tied into the brain's physiological regulation of our bodies, are also linked to the brain's emotional/limbic pleasure-pain center and the instinctual brainstem's sense of distress.

Earlier, our memory of a lemon experience helped us envision an imaginary scene that had a quick and potent effect upon physiological responses. If a lemon memory can do this for us, what does a powerful emotional memory do? How would our subconscious memories of trouble, distress, and pain influence the body's physiology?

The Placebo: An Endorphin Clue

To consider these questions further, let's follow yet another thread of Endorphin evidence which may help to clarify our understanding about the connection between imagery and our physical responses, such as pain. This clue is the phenomenon known as the *placebo effect*. Sometimes, within a hospital setting, doctors and nurses have difficulty helping a patient to receive pain relief. Various pain-killers, including strong narcotics, are tried, but the pain remains. It is in such cases that a placebo is often prescribed. When the placebo effect works, a seemingly useless sugar pill or saline injection amazingly provides pain relief.

The placebo effect has puzzled those who have watched it relieve pain. For many years, this effect has been attributed to a strange psychological quirk within the patient. It has been reasoned that if a sugar pill can provide pain relief, the pain must have existed only psychologically. According to this reasoning, such a psychological problem also could be the reason that traditional, real pain-killers like aspirin or morphine would not relieve these kinds of pain.

Also, many doctors and nurses make a clear distinction between a real pain that has an obvious origin and an "imaginary" pain for which no cause has been found. When a sugar-pill placebo works to relieve this kind of pain, the misconception about imaginary pain is magnified; as though the supposedly non-existent pain-relief of the placebo were further proof that the pain was only imaginary.

Other medical observers have noted that a patient's belief in a given therapeutic method seems to influence the placebo process. Again, the strong emotional component of belief, which indeed causes an internal biochemical response of pain-relief, is often discounted as merely psychological.

But the discovery of intrinsic Endorphins is changing that view. In San Francisco, at the University of California, Dr. Jon Levine and his colleagues have published reports based on a series of experiments which focus upon Endorphin mechanisms and the placebo effect. To do these experiments. Dr. Levine chose patients each of whom was enduring a painful dental procedure. These persons were divided into two groups—those who received pain relief from placebos and those who did not.

As with many Endorphin studies, the opium-antagonist, naloxone, was used throughout these experiments. During the study, a placebo provided significant pain relief, and naloxone consistently reversed this action. Indeed, with naloxone the pain returned and was rated similar to the pain of those who did not obtain relief from the earlier placebo.

In another test, naloxone was used prior to the placebo injection. In this case, naloxone significantly reduced the placebo's capacity to relieve pain. Both of these findings indicate that Endorphins, known to be as intrinsically powerful as morphine, were considered the internal biochemicals relieving the tested pain. Naloxone reversed the placebo effect and also impaired its action. As in many studies before, naloxone indirectly points to the existence of Endorphins and their pain-relieving capacity. These findings bring more evidence to the already established data that placebos often provide consistent, real results.

In our own explorations, we already have wondered about the pains and distresses that are "just in the head." And we can continue to link Endorphin research with an understanding that blends biochemical action with psychological perception. In a 1981 issue of the *American Journal of Nursing*, Samuel Perry, a professor of psychiatry, and George Heidrich, a nurse-researcher, give us even better clues with a thorough review of the placebo effect.

In this article, the authors cite much data that disprove placebo misconceptions. Through this information, placebos are given a broader capacity beyond the relief of questionable pain. Placebos are known to affect significantly such physiological evidence as changes in heartbeat, blood pressure, breathing, blood-cell and chemistry counts, digestive disorders, and immune responses. Sound familiar? Placebos relieve pain, placebos affect systems throughout our bodies. The evidence for a placebo/Endorphin mechanism grows.

If placebo action is indeed a clue that Endorphin mechanisms work throughout the body, other questions quickly arise. How is it that the placebo effect is triggered in the first place? What occurs to trigger the Endorphin process in a placebo situation?

Observations about this phenomenon consistently have linked belief and attitude to the workings of placebos. And, if belief can relieve pain, then an emotional or instinctual distress memory can produce pain through a biochemical process in which Endorphins may well be involved. To be sure, the misconceptions about placebos and pain may be considered simply misinformed assumptions about the process of belief and its effect upon our physiology.

As data about placebos increasingly become evident, placebo action can no longer be limited to a few emotionally troubled patients with imaginary pain.

Placebos provide wide-ranging, positive results in a broad cross-section of age groups, genders, psychological profiles, and clinical situations. By better understanding the placebo effect and its biochemical Endorphin correlation, we can implicate further the potential power of belief, attitude, and perception to affect the quality of our health.

Can We Trigger Endorphins?

As we set out to explore new possibilities for our lives, we have come to realize that Endorphins biochemically influence our bodies, minds, emotions, and thus, our attitudes, perceptions, and even our beliefs.

Now that we know this, we can easily find ourselves asking if we can trigger our Endorphins to improve our life and sense of well-being. Wouldn't it be wonderful if we could do this—wonderful if we could consciously trigger our ongoing Endorphin responses?

The pleasure from Endorphins gives us the desire to explore life's possibilities. In an ongoing way, Endorphins give us the biochemical (including mental and emotional) motivations we need to perceive, reflect, and adapt with flexible responses to our changing environment. Endorphins flow naturally for us. Perhaps then, we should rephrase our question. What stops or limits our natural Endorphin flow?

Endorphins are bio-electrical transmitters of energy—the flow of stimulus to and from the brain.

When we adapt to life's stimulus, even when adaptation takes the form of a rigid sense of structure or belief, we limit our natural capacity to go with the flow of new stimulus. (This is, of course, an irony because Endorphins have influenced us to adapt, in the first place.) But now, as we have adapted too well, we also long for the fresh stimulus of feeling alive.

When someone stops questioning and starts to believe that they've experienced everything, or that there is no longer a sense of freshness about life, the physical support for life follows that belief. The current of Endorphin flow and balance becomes more and more limited. The flame of ongoing bio-electrical synapses starts to die away. But we, who still ask, want to know how to continue to feel life's happiness and well-being.

❊ ❊ ❊

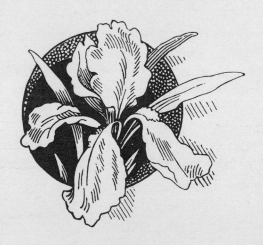

HOW-TO EXPLORATIONS TO TRY

—As you find yourself addicted to eustress, take special note of the difference between eustress and distress in your life. The burnout observed in many stressful occupations is, in part, due to the fine line between eustress and distress. When you feel this kind of burnout, focus on stimulus of the opposite, parasympathetic, resting mode. Smile, laugh, listen to music—develop ways to encourage the relaxation-response in yourself.

—If you are over-stressed, feel a constant sense of distress, or know that you are pushing the sympathetic mode toward workaholism, diversify your activities. If you need to stay active while relaxing, try gardening or another non-competitive outdoor activity. For a relaxation exercise, practice yoga or similar meditation techniques that encourage integration of a peaceful mind and body.

—Deep-breathing exercises have long been a technique for relaxation and heightened awareness. There are Endorphin keyholes throughout your lungs. While sitting quietly, focus on your breathing, consciously aware of inhaling, then exhaling, deeply, and slowly. This is especially useful for encouraging sleep.

—When you are plagued with guilt over the past, or worry about the future, you have become addicted to the biochemistry of these mental activities. Discipline your mind to attend to the present moment. As you do this, use the analogy of tuning into a radio station. Tune your mind away from the addictive static of guilt, worry, and fear—and center it on the clearest reception—focus on the present moment and its experience. As Dr. Fiore has suggested, you are capable—in the powerful present moment—of attending to all of life's challenges *as they arise*, but not before, or after.

—Dreams are a window into the imagery of the unconscious mind—reflecting the biochemistry of the limbic and reptilian brains. Pay attention to the content of your dreams, especially those of conflict. Keep a record of them, thus bringing your unconscious issues into your waking consciousness. Through this technique, you can understand yourself better and begin to resolve the conflicts between these three layers of your brain.

—Recently, the fad of "hugging therapy" has become popular. Hugging has been given credit as a cure-all for many troubles and ills. Hugging sends messages of love, support, and acceptance to the emotional, limbic brain. Hugging may well be an Endorphin trigger. Allow yourself hugs and give them as much as possible—staying comfortable and genuine.

—Take note of the placebo response as you observe it in yourself and others. Have you ever noticed how one person with a positive attitude can uplift an atmosphere? Likewise, a negative attitude can be detrimental to an environment. Use the following impression for positive effect. For instance, smiling can be considered a placebo for yourself and others. Through the act of smiling, the tiny muscles and nerves of your face send biochemical messages back to your brain—saying that you are happy and feeling good. Of course, smiling is contagious—helping others to send to their own brains the same biochemical, euphoric message.

❋ ❋ ❋

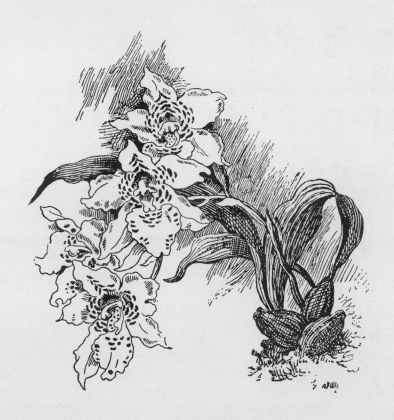

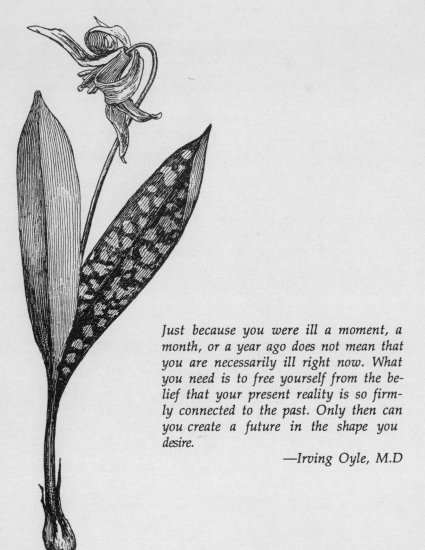

Just because you were ill a moment, a month, or a year ago does not mean that you are necessarily ill right now. What you need is to free yourself from the belief that your present reality is so firmly connected to the past. Only then can you create a future in the shape you desire.

—*Irving Oyle, M.D*

— Four —

Exploring Stimulus
And Change

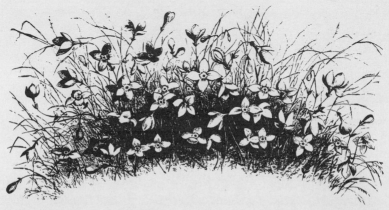

$\mathcal{A}$s we have learned in previous chapters, biochemistry flows to influence our health and happiness—maintaining our bodies, affecting the workings of our minds and emotions, and, thus, our attitudes. A delicate balance of these biochemicals defines our response to stress. Endorphins, working to help the body maintain its balance, are involved in mental and emotional perception of distress or eustress.

When we find ourselves in the darkness of despair and hopelessness, we remember and long for the flash of biochemical eustress again. When there is distress, what triggers the flash of the biochemical, electrical bliss of eustress? We are asking potent questions for ourselves. We know we can have powerful, pleasure-giving biochemicals which bring quality and health into our lives. And, with the addict, we long and ask. How do we trigger the Endorphin response when we need to so desperately?

Perhaps we can recall a past and beautiful time when we were high on life. That powerful memory may have sustained the high for a long time. But now, only the longing remains. Have we only learned to trigger the flash of euphoric biochemicals with memory?

When pain wracks our sense of being, what delivers ease and freedom from pain, again? And, when we are happy, reverberating with the flash of euphoric biochemicals, what keeps the flow of eustress recirculating? Or, what keeps us from a present joy? Do powerful memory biochemicals literally block the flow of incoming stimulus and appreciation, robbing us of a fresh awareness? When we rely on the past, today is not as good as yesterday. Today's potential euphoria is lost in the burden of the longing for yesterday.

In contrast, a child personifies an expectant perspective, alive to interact with the eustress of incoming stimulus. In childhood, life is new. We, as adults, might feel tempted to experience this newness vicariously through the eyes of children who naturally live the joy of life. We forget that we can lengthen the Endorphin cascade by using our own sense of childlike wonder to maintain an ever-present stream of vitality and enthusiasm for being alive, to stay in love with life, ourselves.

Experimenting with Enrichment

To further explore these ideas and some brain research findings that add to our discoveries, let's take an imaginary journey to the University of California at Berkeley. Come, if you will, to the campus, to the neuroscience building, just as the sun comes up. Here we will visit another laboratory where rats are being studied. Dr. Marian Diamond and her colleagues have designed this research setting where they are systematically noting the effect that environments have upon the weight and structure of the brain. Dr. Diamond is comparing brains which are products of variable environments.

Upon entering the room, we might expect to find boring little cages with the rats cooped up, perhaps sleeping, perhaps munching on a bit of food, perhaps exploring a barren cage for the millionth time, waiting for some event that never comes.

But, here, some of the cages are far different from our expectations. In fact, we noticed an unusual noise just as we walked through the door, and we can hear, from a large cage prominently placed on the shelf, a flurry of activity. We notice that this cage has several animals in it. But there is no sense of crowding or density. Here, a group of rats are interacting with each other, seemingly playful and youthful. Several are exploring objects that look like toys. Others climb elaborate stairs and run upon interesting wheels. All seem to be having fun with each other, as though they were families playing together in a utopian environment.

Other cages, standing near, are just as we had expected. Rats lie isolated from one another, each in his own cage. They seem deprived, although they have adequate food, water, light, and air. In one cage, placed beside the large one, a solitary rat sits on his running wheel and watches the proceedings. He seems fascinated by the activity next door, rarely taking his attention from the experiences the lucky rats are having in the next cage.

This laboratory is experimenting with enriched environments. Do toys, friends, family, and new experiences have an effect upon the brain and its biochemical processes? This cage is filled with enrichment, such as toys and special wheels, because of a unique experimental design. Toys are given to the animals to observe how they will interact and what kind of brain response this activity might develop.

Further, new toys are added every few days and old ones replaced. The new playthings differ in size, shape, and design. Thus the experimental environment changes its potential for interaction in an ongoing way.

This research goes beyond simple observations of active rats in "enriched" cages. Observation is just the beginning of an experiment that also has asked— how has enrichment affected their brains? Here Dr. Diamond's research data hold important clues for our own study of the flow of brain biochemicals and Endorphins and of their ongoing impact upon the quality of the health and happiness we seek.

After these enrichment experiments had been completed, the brains of the animals were compared with the brains of rats who had not experienced enrichment. Brain weight was measured and found to be significantly higher in rats who had interacted within an enrichment setting. What does this increased brain weight represent?

To answer this question, let's again focus upon the brain's cellular structure. As we learned in Chapter One, our brains are composed of specialized cells called neurons found within the brain, spinal cord, and peripheral nerve tracts throughout the body. Scientific findings have told us that most neurons do not regenerate. We are born with a certain, fixed number of neurons. This number is the amount we have available to use. In a lifetime, almost no additional nerve cells are created. This finding seems discouraging, perhaps. No new neurons? We would seem to be locked into the brain given us at birth. From this finding, potential for brain growth seems blocked before it even begins.

As you'll recall, the minute branching structures found at the end of each neuron are called dendrites. Every neuron contains this branching system. Close observation of these dendrites shows how neurons can vary from brain to brain. Recalling our tree analogy from Chapter One, we can envision that our neurons are like the limbs of a mature tree. When once a major limb is broken, a new one isn't easily replaced. But, the tree's leaves are like the density of dendrites, potentially changing and regenerating with the seasons. Thus, a densely packed foliage of neuronal dendrites fills the biochemical and electrical bath harbored within our brains.

Herein lies a difference accountable for the variations in brain weight and brain complexity. Within each neuron, itself, dendrite growth is the brain's true potential. Even though we have only a fixed amount of neurons, dendrite branching, stretching, and reaching can continue in an ongoing pattern throughout our lives. It is this growth and increasing density of dendrites, along with the structures which support them, that add the brain weight discovered in Dr. Diamond's enriched animals.

The laboratory rats who have experienced new toys and a community of friends and family develop heavier brains than those who live in solitary cages. The branching growth of their dendrites becomes more dense as these enriched rats interact with a changing environment. The brains of rats who have been confined to changeless, solitary cages have fewer dendrites.

Within the vast harbor of our brains, these seemingly countless, tiny dendrites interact with one another. This neuronal interaction initiates the brain biochemicals about which we have learned so much. Thus, round and about these neurons and their dendrite branches, a continual bath of fluctuating biochemicals emerges, blends and flows. Since we know that the interaction between one dendrite and another gives birth to the brain's electrical process, we thus can consider that an increase in dendrites significantly improves the flow of brain biochemicals. Environmental enrichment then becomes a key to influencing the improvement of a biochemical flow in general and Endorphins in particular.

This concept of enriched environment is now being studied extensively. It is well known that environments which add to an experience have a positive effect upon our brains. Children reared in homes with learning playthings and supportive parents do better in school and adjust better to life; whereas isolated children who have been deprived of attention and interaction with toys and experience show a lessened ability to pay attention, learn, and become successfully involved in life.

Another example comes from Ashley Montagu's book, *Touching, The Human Significance of Skin*. Dr. Montagu cites an example of children who were orphaned and deprived of early human contact. They exhibited a syndrome termed "failure to thrive." Although receiving adequate food and water, their mental and emotional development was retarded. This underscores the significance of environmental stimulus not only within the development of a child but within the adult, as well.

Dr. Diamond's research adds a new dimension to the enriched environment as it applies to adults. Look again at the amusement cage in the Berkeley laboratory. The rats seem youthful, energetic, like children at play. Certainly, they behave more youthfully than their solitary counterparts in neighboring cages. Let's check the data sheets documenting the age of these specimens. Eight hundred days? It couldn't be! That would mean that these animals are elderly, even age'd. Most laboratory rats only average six hundred days of life. These, who yet seem so youthful, have lived into very old age, one-third beyond their life expectancy. They remain active and even seem happy in their busy lives. They still seem to benefit physiologically and psychologically from this enriched environment.

Dr. Diamond's research focuses upon aging—but not in the common, discouraging studies about disease and infirmity. Her work centers upon increasing the lifespans of experimental animals. Through this focus, enriched environments are studied as major comparative factors in brain development and life maintenance. As a result, Dr. Diamond and her colleagues have been able to increase laboratory lifespans up to nine-hundred days, fifty percent longer than the original figure for elderly rats of six hundred. Do these rats have more to live for and thus live longer? Dr. Diamond's Berkeley laboratory takes that question seriously.

From what is generally known about the importance of early childhood development, we could expect that these enriched rats are successful in their interaction with toys and each other because they have been so conditioned in their youth. But here, Dr. Diamond adds an additional twist to the experimental design. These rats, although they are now eight-hundred-days old, have only recently been introduced to this enriched environment.

At the elderly age of six-hundred days, they were taken from the solitary environments in which they were raised and placed in a cage with toys and

friends. (We could speculate upon the brain processes of the seemingly wistful solitary rat next door.)
Like the previous, younger rats, the elderly enriched
rats interacted actively, climbing upon structures and
playing with the new toys that recently had been
added to the cage. We know that we humans are
sometimes socially conditioned to believe that when
we become elderly, we also become inactive. But,
these rats apparently had not received a previous
conditioning. They simply interacted in "today's"
cage. Such an environment seems enriched to
nurture life and to sustain its sense of quality.

Dr. Diamond's experimental design also is
unique in that her animals are not sacrificed at a
specified time in the study. After the natural time of
death, the enriched rat brains are studied in comparison with the brains of rats who died in solitary
cages. These findings of increased brain weight and
corresponding dendrite density are beginning clues
about the lengthening and increasing quality of life;
beginning answers to our own questions about how
these enrichment studies might apply to us.

In a 1982 lecture at the University of California,
San Francisco, Dr. Diamond discussed these findings.
She wondered if we could directly correlate the dendrite growth of enriched rats' brains to the human
brain. "Why not?" she asked. A neuron is a basic
building block for all brains found in living crea-
tures. The comparison between the small brain of a
rat and the larger brain of a human can be likened to
the similarities between a wild flower and a tree.
Both are plants, structured with similar cells, grow-

ing and stretching in response to the environment. One is simply larger and more complex in design than the other.

The Cage Within

Tiny laboratory animals with seemingly simple brains have benefited from the experimental design of cages enriched with goodies. Why wouldn't we—who also have vast dendrite potential for interaction with our own brain biochemicals—also benefit from enriched environments? Indeed, we might find ourselves longing for enrichment, even as the solitary watcher in the neighboring cage seemed wistful in his observation. Our lives sometimes seem like a cage from which we cry out for a new toy or new friend. But this enclosure is a feeling-perception originating within.

As we have learned, a certain blend or imbalance of biochemicals within our brains could reinforce our sensation of being locked into ourselves. Too many Endorphins, or the lack of them, have the potential either to reinforce or create perceptions of distress and pain. We might find ourselves consumed by a biochemical sense of parched longing. We might feel fragile, insignificant, or lost. At times, we might perceive a sense of distance from all who nurture and care for us. Within this potential biochemical imbalance, boredom, inactivity, and solitude could then enclose our lives; we could become, like the lonely watcher in a cage, apart from the enrichment experienced by others.

At other times we can be hindered by our own raging emotions. A storm of biochemical anger or indignation within ourselves can erupt with volcanic force—to sabotage our consciousness from within or to burst forth, overflowing upon the lives of those around us.

Or, we can be swept with tidal waves of guilt, doubt, and self-pity. These self-destructive feelings may eventually submerge anger's volcanic heat, but they also can devastate our consciousness or sense of identity. We can find ourselves imprisoned in our own brain's biochemistry, longing for that enriched environment to enliven us to freedom from a crushing sense of self, while at the same time feeling overwhelmed by the violence and weight of these biochemical onslaughts.

As described in a recent *Discover* article called "The Mind Within The Brain," scientists elaborate on what we already have discovered—that these devastating feelings represent a specific blend of biochemicals arising from within our brains.

From this information, and from what we've already learned about the triune brain layers in Chapters Two and Three, we can surmise that instinctual feelings might well erupt from biochemical dictates toward survival. Our ancestors survived because of their brains' biochemical priorities to fight for the survival of one's kin or herd. Within these instinctual dictates, powerful biochemical forces—yes, even Endorphins—reinforced these survival tides, which seemingly can lock us into the anger, hostility, guilt, and self-pity described earlier. Our destructive emotions can build bars between ourselves and the freedom of life's potential quality.

A Window to Freedom

Let's try imagining again. Picture a hospital corridor, leading to a row of rooms. As we examine the cubicles, they seem very like cages, designed only for efficiency of care. Along this row of rooms, groups of patients, similar in their condition and appearance, are recovering from major surgery. These people have been very ill, requiring the best technology that medical science can give. And now they are slowly recovering, waiting for the healing process to take hold so that they may be discharged from a hospital confinement.

This recovery process, like the distressing emotions we have just explored, also seems like a prison, encasing ill people inside themselves. A row of hospital rooms—like a row of cages—houses physical illness which confines through pain, weakness, nausea—tides of symptoms indicating a disease process. In a recent study about healing, a similar row of hospital rooms was likewise the topic of consideration. In this experiment, rooms were designed to be similar to each other, very like our own earlier imagery. But, within the study's design, some rooms presented a unique difference.

All were small cubicles which housed the sick. But some of the rooms had windows with views to the outside world. Is it possible that the enrichment of a window's view could quicken the recovery process? Would a visual stimulus influence the bio-electrical flow to hasten health? This was the condition which researchers set about to observe, in seeking answers to these questions.

As we could guess from our own experience with Dr. Diamond's enriched rats, those patients who had a view to the outside world did recover faster than those who had no new stimulus within their hospital space. The view, itself, seemed to be the key to a faster recovery. But why? A window view brings enrichment and change to the experience of an ill person, because visual information stimulates neurons and thus influences the balance of brain biochemicals.

Illness is most often a process of recovery. Within many healing processes, symptoms of fevers, weaknesses, pains and aches are simple, yet seemingly disruptive, signs that recovery is progressing. The body fights disease and in many cases wins, despite numerous apparent failures or setbacks. The prisons of illness and distress may be like a long tunnel through which we pass, to find recovery and eustress at the end.

Can we suggest that enriched environments might quicken our sense of freedom from the biochemical tunnels of disease and distress arising from within? Does an enriched environment somehow trigger an Endorphin response, which would then influence the quality of our bio-electrical flow, and thus improve our healing and our potential quality of life?

The Wellspring of Sensory Stimulus

Looking closely again at the brain, we ask what effect does an enriched environment create? Neuron cells—at one recent estimate, ten billion of them within each human brain—contain a vast dendrite potential for experiencing the quality of life. These dendrites stretch, reach, growing toward stimulus, creating and developing in a flow of biochemical electricity, keeping us alive and potentially well.

As dendrites grow and stretch, their edges reach to touch other dendrites from other cells. At this meeting, a synapse happens like a spark of electrical conduction. This process ignites biochemicals within each synaptic gap as a match strikes a fire. Imagine all the synapse flashes from all the meeting dendrite branches. This ball of energy, which is your brain, shining upon the body like the sun upon the earth, floods your physical form, even to your fingers and toes.

Remember again that this ongoing bio-electrical sun within our heads also directly influences our biochemical cascades of energy which regulate our hormone balance, our immune strength, and our health. This is the body's own electricity, influenced by numerous biochemicals, known and unknown, flowing to spark and maintain all aspects of our lives.

124

Stimulus and Change

In a recent brain biochemistry review in the journal *Cellular and Molecular Biology*, Peter Vaughn, a researcher at Glasgow University in Scotland, suggests that some Endorphins may "set the gain" for maintaining our physiology. Taking this analogy from electronics, Dr. Vaughn's concept shows that the Endorphins which function throughout our vast biochemical and bio-electrical network may well be the *regulators* of our health processes. From our own explorations of Endorphin issues, like tolerance/dependence, addiction, depression, distress, eustress, and euphoria, we may be working toward a better understanding about how this regulation takes place.

This vast network is always in a state of flux. Indeed, each of these dendrite synapses fires for only the briefest of moments. When we perceive illness, distress, anger, fear, or longing, our bodies seem to be like unchangeable, concrete prisons. But these seemingly negative biochemical conditions are only a present perception. A biochemical balance can be flushed into the past in the very next moment. New information can impact fully upon our brains at any time through this five-sensory network.

In the case of a patient confined to a hospital cubicle, a view out the window brings new visual information to a brain that also is involved in a bodily strengthening and recovery process. In the case of Dr. Diamond's laboratory rats, dendrites grow and flourish with the stimulus of enrichment. A flush of new synapses ignites biochemicals, influencing the flow of the bio-electrical growth.

To sum up, a hospital room with a stimulating

view is very like the rats' laboratory cage with new toys. In the above study, the recovery process was accelerated by a view to the outside world, an enriched environment to drink in and appreciate. Our brain's bio-electricity, like the bio-electricity of laboratory rats, can be receptive to the enrichment delivered by the electrical stimulus of sensory awareness. Our internal biochemical feeling of imprisonment can be released by a sensory stimulus of enrichment.

Vision, melody, aroma, flavor, texture, and space, all forms of bio-electrical stimulus, are the inputs that bring our brains our own individualized sense of reality. When stimulus changes, biochemistry changes, and with this flow our perception of reality can change, too. As we now know, Endorphins affect this process. In a review of Endorphin sensory systems, A.W. Duggan, a pharmacologist at the Australian National University in Canberra, points to growing evidence that Endorphins are somehow involved in the electrical processing of sensory information. Citing two studies, Dr. Duggan discusses how the specialized Endorphin called *Enkephalin* may influence the vision capacity of the retina and the smelling capacity of the olfactory bulb. Sensory information becomes bio-electrical stimulus, which modifies brain responses.

In research that studies the sense of touch, electrical stimulus seems to initiate the biochemical events resulting in increased Endorphin levels. In one growing branch of Endorphin research, it has been shown that electrical stimulus to the body can relieve pain. As we've learned in Chapter One, many types of electrical devices and designs have been observed to function in this way. Electrodes placed within a specialized area of the brain have produced, when stimulated, significant relief for the chronic and intractable pain of terminal illness. This pain relief is consistently reversed by the Endorphin antagonist, naloxone.

Another use of electrical stimulus common in hospitals and pain clinics today is a portable device which allows a pain patient to place skin electrodes adjacent to the site of pain, and control the electrical stimulus, accordingly. As stimulus is released, pain is usually relieved or minimized.

Acupuncture is another example of stimulus and Endorphin response. In several studies since Endorphins have been discovered, it was found that acupuncture produces pain relief that is later reversed by the Endorphin antagonist, naloxone. But, like the more direct electrical stimulus therapies, the value of acupuncture pain relief seems to fluctuate at times. Why would a stimulus treatment to induce changes in biochemicals, such as Endorphins, have inconsistent results?

An arthritis specialist, Dr. Richard Wold, uses an electrical device placed to stimulate acupuncture points in the treatment of severe arthritis pain. He has remarked that the variable pain relief from these devices, similar to relief from placebos, seems to correlate with *belief* in the electrical treatment's effectiveness. Electrical stimulus triggers an Endorphin response to pain. But belief, another factor in the bio-electrical process, could strengthen or prolong electricity's effectiveness, just as disbelief, yet another bio-electrical event within the brain, can shorten or decrease any kind of therapeutic effectiveness.

One reviewer of Endorphin findings, Dr. D. G. Smyth at the London National Institute for Medical Research, has suggested a similar perspective. Dr. Smyth wonders whether fluctuations in the pain-relief potency of Endorphin action are sensitive to environmental stimulus. Dr. Smyth suggests also that factors such as age, gender, stress, and mental and emotional experiences throughout our lives can influence bio-electrical processes. These factors can be reinforced by education, by our childhood experiences, by the way we've been treated, or by expectations thrust upon us. Again, attitudes, perceptions, and beliefs, molded and reinforced by previous biochemical events, and probably by Endorphins, themselves, can affect such bodily processes as pain, distress, eustress, and healing.

Obstructions in The Stream

Environmental stimulus transmitted through our electrical five-sensory pathway, can deliver enriched information into our brains. As we have noted within the realm of sensation and touch, therapeutic electrical stimulus, such as acupuncture, can relieve pain through an Endorphin mechanism. But, as in cases of variable pain relief and placebos, perceptions and beliefs about the stimulus may affect the outcome of the treatment.

It is as though belief, itself, modifies the balance

of brain biochemistry. Attitudes, perceptions, and conditions previously relegated to the mind would seem to influence a receptivity to stimulus. If someone believes in a treatment, it appears that biochemistry could be affected, accordingly. A lack of belief or blocked perception might well change biochemical environment, as well.

From the preceding information, we can see that the experience of enrichment is not a simple process for healing. Our human sense of enrichment goes beyond new toys or larger cages containing our friends and family. We can and do benefit from enrichment stimulus. But, our own *perception* about the enrichment information being received from our five senses seems to be a key bio-electical factor. Receptivity to enrichment seems to affect the flow of biochemistry and to affect our awareness of enrichment.

How is it that our brains, with infinitely vast dendrite potential, can become so obstructed that we lose our ability to receive the enrichment available to us at any given moment? We live in a beautiful world, filled with opportunities for enriching experiences and relationships. Except in times of confinement (and sometimes, even then), there is always a view to the outside, interesting sounds, intriguing textures, warmth, chill, sweetness, spice. Varying experiences await our awareness in any present moment. Even Helen Keller, whose capacity to receive stimuli was limited to three senses—touch, taste, and smell—felt enriched by her appreciation of a beautiful world.

Potential Influence of Past and Future

We have been considering electrical processes in our study of the brain, its biochemistry, and Endorphins. Would some sort of electrical static be the stimulus obstacle which blocks the receptivity of enriched awareness? We have learned that imagery is brain potential that can be either harmful or helpful to us. Through our ability to envision, we can create biochemical experience within ourselves. Our earlier lemon imagery was an example of this brain capacity.

You'll recall that we could, through simple suggestions to ourselves, envision the sight of a lemon tree, hear a slight breeze, feel the fruit hanging heavy on a branch, sense the bumpy peeling, smell and taste the pungent juice. When we envision in this way, a five-sensory experience may occur as realistically within our biochemistry as though we were truly beside a lemon tree.

Dr. Neil Fiore, who first shared this lemon example with us at a seminar in 1980, explains how this brain potential can be like static, interfering and hindering our awareness.

We have the ability to remember past experience. This our brain can do in detail. In fact, some past experiences seem more vivid now than the present moment which fleets by. This detail, even to the memory of smell, sensation, and feeling, is etched into our brains so strongly that we can relive these experiences again and again.

The famous composer Ludwig van Beethoven was able to use this brain capacity for the improvement of his life. In his last years, he became totally deaf. Yet, his ability to remember and hear sound and harmony in his mind was so effective that he still was able to compose powerful symphonies for others to hear with their ears and to enjoy.

Similarly, our brains have the capacity to envision future experience. We can readily pre-conceive an experience before it happens. We can anticipate the tastes of food while yet reading the recipe from a cookbook. We can plan a vacation in minute detail and fully enjoy this experience, even before the reservations are made. But, past memories or future visions can become literal electrical static within our brain's capacity, interfering with our reception of a bio-electical stimulus in the present moment.

Dr. Fiore has focused on this problem in his stress management classes. He describes how a biochemical potential can be harmful or restrictive in our lives. Through our ability to remember the past, we can plague ourselves with the static of "if only" visions. We can relive painful or bad experiences, turning them round and round in our heads, wishing that these experiences had been different or more pleasing. We can overwhelm ourselves with guilt perception about what we didn't do or should have done in the past. Or, we can maintain the heat of anger, or the ice of resentment, fresh in the brain's biochemistry, blocking our potential in the present moment.

Even beautiful past experiences can rob us of the

present potential for enriched sensory awareness. We can remember nostalgic happiness, back to the times when the world seemed better than it does today. We can relive this past again and again, even to be tricked into believing that past memory is present reality.

We earlier reviewed how Endorphins can be involved in the memory process. When we are happy in a situation, biochemical euphoria bonds that moment within our brains, creating a strong memory. The Endorphin researchers we met in Chapter Three, Drs. Larry Stein and James D. Belluzzi, of the University of California at Irvine, speculate that Endorphins could be the specific brain biochemicals which achieve this brain process.

When we experience happiness or euphoria, a biochemical occurrence reinforces the memory, perhaps to etch a moment's bliss into our very dendrites and neurons. Through this process, past experience may be conjured up again and again in the seeking after a biochemical "high."

Dr. Fiore also warns of another potential problem in the brain's ability to envision future experience. We can distress ourselves with the static of "what if" visions. This is where worry and fear can influence our biochemistry. Dr. Fiore shares examples of students who inadvertently use this envisioning to sabotage their learning. They might say "what if I fail this exam!" or "what if I'm kicked out of school!" This worry imagery is an inappropriate and distressing use of brain ability.

Worry and fear are distress signals—bio-electrical

static which can, if allowed to be chronic, affect on-going bodily processes.

You'll remember that stress, itself, is a known trigger of the Endorphin response. Is it possible then that a sense of worry or fear could create the stress that induces Endorphin bio-electicity? If this is the case, a chronic use of worry-imagery or fear-envisioning could be addictive, triggering the tolerance/dependence cycle we have studied in past chapters.

If we literally can become biochemically addicted to fear or worry static, accumulating stress to a distressing level, we can thus easily harm ourselves in a way similar to the heroin addict who becomes dependent upon destructive choices and behaviors.

As with enjoyment of biochemical nostalgia, envisioning a future happiness can also be the static which blocks the enriched potential of our present awareness. We might spend a large amount of bio-electrical energy wishing for that far-off day when we can live happily ever after. We think about how our situation might be different or about a wonderful relationship we could have, or about next year's vacation, or retirement in a decade. It is good to have the biochemical capacity to plan for the future or correct past mistakes. But when this envisioning becomes chronic, it gives us a false sense of reality. Future and past imagery only *seem* to be the present experience.

In this inappropriate reality, we can encumber ourselves—again, like the addict who maintains a baseline dose of a drug, but soon needs a greater "fix."

If we maintain a baseline happiness on yesterday's nostalgia or the future's promise, we can soon find ourselves longing for a greater euphoria. Our addictions to memory or anticipation block our potential to experience today's fresh impetus; the powerful euphoric biochemistry which the present moment brings.

Based upon preconceived attitudes or upon the interference of worry, fear, doubt, or guilt, we can resist a positive and electrically euphoric response to the stimulus of change. If and when we resist change, and especially as we grow older, we may block the stimulus potential for our brains to remain capable of maintaining or regulating the quality of our health and life. Just as belief in, and receptivity to, stimulus might positively influence bio-electical events, so might stubborn resistance be the ultimate negative static which blocks and stagnates a fresh bio-chemical flow.

What causes resistance to change? We have within our consciousness a feeling for what our world is like. In this way, our environment might seem to be quite structured and safe. We might then learn to rely upon this sense of structure for the sake of stability and constancy in our sense of identity. We generally accept that one season flows into another, that eventually, generations flow one to another. But today, in this present moment, conditions often feel permanent and thus, reliable. This awareness or definition of the world as a structured place is a conditioned way of perceiving. This idea may be the concept which we have been taught to believe and trust. Biochemically, we have noted that these beliefs are reinforced by a bio-electical process which seems to etch itself into our brains. We come to rely upon our environment as an unchanging, structured place to be.

Thus, we might find ourselves resisting the novel, changing, and incredibly enriching environment of today's world. We might even find ourselves wishing for a quiet, solitary cage in which to hibernate.

Change: The Flow Widens

Return now to the enriched rat cage in Berkeley to examine one of the most important aspects of Dr. Diamond's study of brain responses. Another few days have passed and the cage looks somehow different. The same sense of enrichment remains, but something new has been added. Before, the rats were running on wheels, climbing stairs, and playing with toys, now they seem to be busy with a new set of objects. This they seem to do with relish, keeping up a level of interest and activity far different from those rats who live in cages without playthings. As before, they are very active, with the eager activity of exploration that allows them to interact with today's environment.

In these experiments, deliberate change of toys is an ongoing stimulus for exploration and interaction. Dr. Diamond has explained that this aspect of her enrichment design is very significant and may hold the key to the *longevity* her laboratory animals have been able to achieve. As the "enriched" cage receives new toys and the used playthings are removed, the experimental environment changes and encourages the animals to maintain an explorative response to newness.

Dr. R. J. Katz, a mental health researcher at the University of Michigan Medical Center, has considered the connection between exploration and Endorphins. In a letter to the editor of the *Journal of Theoretical Biology*, Dr. Katz suggests that Endorphins, themselves, are involved in reinforcing the explorative and enthusiastic behavior we have been learning about. He cites examples of laboratory animals increasing their cage exploration when Endorphins are artificially induced. This finding strongly indicates that Endorphins are biochemicals which support the life-maintenance behavior of exploration, foraging, and seeking to interact with an environment.

But Dr. Katz investigates beyond an artificial dose of Endorphins to study exploration. In a review of his own research, Dr. Katz explains how naloxone, again acting as an Endorphin antagonist, can diminish explorative responses, even in a novel or enriched environment.

From these concepts, we can readily suggest that Endorphins reinforce an explorative response to an enriched environment, and naloxone subverts this response. Can we also suggest that exploration, in turn, reinforces the Endorphin response? Let's take a clue from these experiments to do some exploring of our own.

We have discovered a key factor in the enriched laboratory environment. This is the ingredient of change. The laboratory animals maintained highly active, exploratory responses to a changing environment. Their brains seemed to benefit from this stimulus of change. Dendrites stretched and grew, creating more potential for synapses with other dendrites. More synapses, more flashes of bio-electricity, and the brain remains ablaze with electrical life. Change, stimulus, explorative response—an ongoing process affects the quality and longevity of life.

As we know, Dr. Diamond's enriched and exploring rats at the Berkeley laboratory lived longer, stayed healthier, and remained more active than those who were deprived of the stimulus of change. How can we give ourselves the perception that Dr. Diamond's rats received? How can we condition ourselves to be more receptive to the inevitable change that we find ourselves meeting each day?

Today, scientists look seriously at change, itself, as a topic of consideration. Indeed, the Nobel Prize has been awarded for such studies. One recipient, Ilya Prigogine, is a chemist from Belgium. Dr. Prigogine began his study of change by observing the nature of complex chemical reactions, the basic processes of life. Watching these interactions, Dr. Prigogine notes that, as chemical reactions combine or separate, these events are universally accompanied by the presence of turbulence or what he terms *chaos*.

Dr. Prigogine then theorizes about the inherent

value of this turbulence or chaos. He sees chaos as a fermenting process which acts to restructure chemicals in the process of change, like a necessary catalyst for life's growth. Further, Dr. Prigogine notes that the more complex the chemical, the greater the turbulence of change, or of chaos during change.

How would this apply to our own studies of how change can affect us? When we perceive change as a threat, we begin to resist its flow. But, the more we resist this seeming chaos, the more complex the turbulence problem becomes. (And the potential for distress and subsequent disease increases.)

However, Dr. Prigogine theorizes that chaos, itself, (as in the world today) is an essential prelude to all growth or improvement of structure in any form. Rather than being worried or fearful about this chaos, Dr. Prigogine is optimistic about this phenomenon. He sees in his observations a paradigm shift toward the concept that all living systems continue on a fluctuating journey through an ever-changing environment.

This organization and reorganization is a continuous cycle of energy exchange observed not only within chemical solutions, but within human beings, societies, and the very fabric of nature, itself. This seeming randomness is simply moving from an old order, through chaos, to a higher order of organization. Indeed, Dr. Prigogine paradoxically implies that structure, seemingly "fixed" to our perspective, is really change in slow motion. Dr. John Hughes, one of the first Endorphin researchers, has remarked that Endorphins are a notable example of how our bodies flexibly adapt moment by moment to ongoing biological events. Endorphins enable us to respond to our changing environment in a positive, euphoric, life-sustaining way. This observation about Endorphins also underscores Dr. Prigogine's theories about life and change.

If we can make a shift in consciousness for ourselves, especially remembering the value a changing environment had for laboratory rats, we might be able to adopt Dr. Prigogine's optimism about change. As we have discovered in our explorations before, researchers are also viewing brain processes in the same way that Dr. Prigogine sees life. Our brains are not fixed, unchangeable structures, but harbors for the fluctuating flow of bio-electicity, an infinitely complex process for the ongoing maintenance of life.

Euphoria—The Motive
Toward Change

In Dr. Diamond's work, a changing environment seemed the enriched catalyst for improved brain development, dendrite growth, and longevity. Through dendrite interaction, synaptic activity releases brain biochemicals. Could the existence of a changing environment be the stressful catalyst which ignites the euphoric potential of Endorphins? Do extra or more consistent Endorphins flow in the brains of laboratory animals who seem to enjoy their play, their changing toys, and each other? Does the ongoing flow of Endorphins have anything to do with the longevity which these animals have achieved? Does our concept of enrichment really point to an environment which can somehow, through change, trigger an ongoing, consistent Endorphin eustress response which could keep us feeling well and happy? Consider the possibility that enriched environments do stimulate Endorphins and the bio-electical quality of life. We know that stimulus can produce Endorphins. Such a stimulus, known to work through the sense of touch, can literally relieve pain. Endorphin responses come from stimulus to our other four senses, like visions, sounds, tastes, and smells.

We have also explored the possibility that beliefs, attitudes, and perceptions can have a significant influence upon the electrical factors in these biochemical processes. Belief can modify and even provide, as in the case of placebo pain relief, an Endorphin response. It would follow then, that attitude also could influence any incoming electrical sensation toward Endorphin production and the awareness of euphoria or distress. Is our reality enriched or deprived because of our bio-electrical perception that it is so?

Imagine again; this time find yourself in the enriched environment of a mountainside forested with some of the tallest trees on earth. Upon this steep range there once walked a man who seemed pale, breathless, distressed, and diseased, from tuberculosis. During our envisioning, we will learn about this man who was named Galen Clark. His story began in 1856. As we follow the events of this true account, we will be exploring another example of enrichment's role in healing and the improvement of life's quality.

Our mountainside includes the vast and beautiful region of Yosemite, California. Galen Clark had lived most of his early life enduring successive financial failures. Already a widower and destitute, he couldn't support his children, for he was stricken with tuberculosis. His physicians had already told Galen that this condition was terminal, that his lungs had sustained irreversible damage, and that his last days would be filled with suffering, pain, and breathlessness.

Because of this woeful pronouncement and a frightfully bloody cough which seemed to show that his death was imminent, Galen Clark decided to spend his last days traveling to a beautiful place he had briefly visited earlier in his life. He arranged for his children to be fostered, bid farewell to his old existence, and took his diseased body to Yosemite.

Despite his earlier encounter, Galen was unprepared for the magnificent scenery and new experience that greeted him. He settled on the western slope of the Yosemite Sierra, waiting to die in this forested paradise. But as the days passed, his energy returned, and he found himself walking up and down the steep forest slopes with greater ease of breath and stamina.

He took a great interest in the Yosemite Valley, almost a day's hard hike away. And, closer to his own camp, Galen Clark discovered the great Sequoia trees in what is now called the Mariposa Grove. In tending the needs of these great trees, and guarding them from potential exploitation, his dedication was such that he was appointed, in 1866, the first official guardian of Yosemite, ten years beyond his death sentence. Galen Clark intermittently held that post and its active, stressful but enriching responsibilities for another forty years, dying in old age at ninety-six.

Galen Clark found enrichment, healing, and happiness by choosing to interact with change in a challenging and beautiful environment. Were his physicians incorrect in their earlier grim prognosis? Probably not. But how did Galen Clark's body, stricken with the advanced disease changes of tuberculosis, return to the condition of vigor which allowed him to lead an extremely active life for another fifty years?

We cannot know for sure. But likely, it was a convergence of factors—clear air, increased exercise, the exhilaration and eustress of new and changing endeavor, the appreciation of nature's beauty, the new-found expectation and love of life—all of which are potential stimulus triggers—that helped to re-create a healing flow within his diseased body. Perhaps even more important than healing—but perhaps significant to his recovery—were his happiness and deep fulfillment in his new life.

An enriched environment, which we can further explore, stimulates dendrite branching and growth, creating euphoria biochemicals which impact upon our health and happiness.

Thus, our bio-electrical river runs, affecting every moment of our lives. Indeed, it seems to affect all that we do, think, and feel. It reflects our consciousness, our perceptions, our ideas about ourselves and others. Biochemistry affects our awareness, our actions, our minds, and our bodies. It affects what our five senses communicate to our brains; it affects the messages which flow to our bodies to feel pain or pleasure, stress, distress or eustress, to experience disease or health. All of these factors flow together within the tiny, subtle, yet powerful, realm of the brain's electricity.

We have thus far explored some of the provocative research and laboratory experiments that have lead to Endorphin clues. Upon discovering Endorphin concepts, researchers look back on what they've recently learned and thus suggest concepts for future study.

From our own experience and experiment with life, we can likewise consider how these ideas may affect us personally; we can develop a new focus upon the present and future enrichment of our lives. Euphoric, health-maintaining Endorphins, with vast potential for the enhancement of life's quality, can be studied with a view to our own possibilities.

❋ ❋ ❋

HOW-TO EXPLORATIONS TO TRY

—What does an "enriched" environment mean to you? As you develop your own ongoing definition, remember that diversity and change are key ingredients, like spice in a recipe. As much as possible, keep yourself receptive to your changing world. As you become receptive to the ongoing stimulus of the present moment, this stimulus will encourage your brain's dendrite growth—enabling you to interact with your environment and life more effectively.

—When you find yourself unreceptive or "bogged down" in an environment that once gave you joy, find ways to bring fresh stimulus to the setting—perhaps a vase of flowers, or different music. Remember that most man-made environments tend to be static or unchanging—their quality is dependent upon what we can bring to them in the form of our beliefs and attitudes.

—When you hear yourself say "what if?" you are using your capability to envision and plan for the future. But if you use this ability for chronic worry or fear, you may be addicted to the kind of stress which can easily lead to distress and disease. To help yourself stop this detrimental cycle, deliberately replace worry images with attuned focus on the present moment, its beauties, needs, and potentials.

—When you catch yourself reliving the past, you are using the "re-play" capability of your brain's biochemistry. Especially if your past seems better than today, it's tempting to live in a memory of the past.

144

But past memories do not stimulate dendrite growth and the electrical flow of fresh biochemistry. Only a focused receptivity to present stimulus can do that. As much as possible, switch from the "re-play" to the real game.

—Sometimes, life does seem filled with problems or troubles that are overwhelming. Then, it is even easier to become addicted to worrying about the future or remembering a seemingly better past. However, the solution to the problem you might perceive often lies within your own potential to grow in response to change. As you interact with life, dendrite growth creates new synapses and the flow of fresh brain biochemistry. These changes in your brain can help you to cope more effectively with troubles as they arise.

—When you feel imprisoned in one mode of feeling or being, especially if you're feeling negative or overwhelmed, try receiving a full-body massage or foot rub. The skin is filled with Endorphin receptors, thus—massage, acupressure, foot reflexology, and other forms of "body work" are a potent pain-relief stimulus through the sense of touch. These therapies also can help to release biochemicals necessary for a change of perception.

—As you seek your own growth through an ongoing interaction with life, consider opinions and beliefs that may be different from your own. Look for alternative belief systems that might well have a positive effect upon your problem. Through open consideration, your own growing dendrites and synapses can incorporate what you are learning into what you already know. Examine your belief systems—especially where you have disbelief. Remembering that belief is a bio-electrical process that can be influenced for change, keep your mind receptive to new stimulus, new ideas, and new options.

—Consider the beauty of nature as the ultimate enriched environment—an ongoing, potent Endorphin trigger. Like Galen Clark, allow yourself to be in nature as much as possible. Take your break from work in a garden or park. Plan your vacations around seeing beautiful nature areas. Once there, don't just look; involve your other four senses, interact with your environment.

❊ ❊ ❊

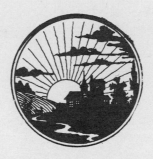

I have discovered that I also live in creation's dawn, the morning stars still sing together, and the world, not yet half made, becomes more beautiful every day.
                                                    —John Muir

— Five —

Happiness And Healing From Within

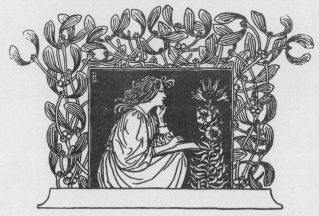

*H*ow special any day can be! In a review of our recent past, we can look back to remember a chain of extraordinary moments that glisten like gold in a rushing stream. These times burn in our memories, strung like glowing beads on the chain of otherwise forgotten days and years.

Consider what gave these times their preciousness, their heightened awareness—a sensory freshness, a new experience, a moment of profound inspiration. We may have felt a chill of sudden perception down the spine, or a surge of commitment to loving, giving, and receiving. These times seem to have a reality outside of space and time. Endorphins? Yet another facet of biochemical influences to ponder. Is it possible that during times of most profound love and joy our brains are brimming full of the biochemicals of euphoria?

Following The Flow
from Being to Becoming

We are constantly ablaze with bio-electricity, a flow of glistening energy, a shining sphere, created and recreated, to be created again. Infinite in variety and complexity, infinitesimal in size but powerful in impact, our biochemistry maintains the homeostasis of our health and the feeling called happiness.

As detailed in Karl Pribram's holographic brain theory that was reviewed in Chapter One, the brain's energy field is like a three-dimensional camera, receiving information in the form of images. Look carefully at an object in front of you, then close your eyes and remember that object. Your brain receives visual information and then records it as memory. Both are examples of the holographic imagery which the brain's biochemical energy field maintains.

Remember also that this imagery is more than the visual receiving and recording of objects in front of your eyes. This imagery is multi-sensory, simultaneously recording the sounds, sensations, tastes, and smells which combine with vision to create what is called experience. And then, this multi-sensory brain experience is recorded, to be placed in memory and the stream called consciousness.

Then, as life flows from one moment to the next,

established consciousness interacts with present experience to define our multi-sensory imagery in the present moment, and our ongoing perceptions, beliefs, and attitudes to life.

But, what affects the flow toward the experience we call health and the consciousness we call happiness? In Chapter Four, we learned of Ilya Prigogine's theory that life is defined by change. In his view, which both includes and widens beyond the body's functioning, all nature is a process which flows from states of being to states of becoming. In this concept, life is more than the fixed moment it may seem to be. Being is constantly becoming within each moment in time, to be changed again, and yet again.

Our own exploration through streams of bioelectrical consciousness helps us to understand this simple and yet seemingly complex theory. Time flows in a stream from past, through present, to future, which then becomes present, then past—eternally. In terms of our conscious awareness of time, reality is composed of both being and becoming—combining to reflect the experience and consciousness of today, from moment to moment. Both are necessary. Today is a product of yesterday's being, flowing through becoming. If being is without becoming, the future will be just another outworn version of today. If becoming is without being, however, the present awareness is lost. Like parasympathetic and sympathetic, both being and becoming work together to balance each other toward a quality life each day.

Brain biochemistry flows in the same pattern,

except that time is measured in seconds instead of days. Our present moment of being is experience, which has streamed from the past moment's becoming. In the future, a few seconds away, our being is again becoming. Thus, the brain's electrical biochemistry sustains the ongoing experience and consciousness we call life. Let's explore how this changing flow from being to becoming can optimize our health and happiness.

We have investigated the scientist's world of laboratory experiment. Rats living in cages and enriched by a changing, social environment live longer, remain more active, and have brain growth reflecting this environment. The dendrites in the brains of these rats branch more densely, interacting with one another to ignite potential euphoric synapses. This continual electrical and biochemical flow supports all of the brain's activities.

We have learned how, in a laboratory environment, enrichment affects dendrite growth and the flow of bio-electrical life. We have explored many facets of Endorphin research and pondered how the threads of this exploration might apply to our own health and life. As we begin now to weave these threads into a pattern of meaning, let's expand the concept of enrichment beyond a cage filled with new toys. What indeed is the enrichment that can so beneficially affect our brains, our dendrite growth, our own flow of biochemical support of life? And, what about the family called Endorphins? In some way, the environment within which we live and perceive can enrich the flow of Endorphins. But how?

An Experiment in Healing

Let's begin to define what our own enrichment might be with the story of a man who became his own experiment in the regaining of health and the improvement of life's quality. As described in his book, *The Anatomy of An Illness*, which recently became a television movie, Norman Cousins relates how he became deathly ill from a rare connective-tissue disease. He was devastated by the pronouncement that his disease was incurable, terminal, and would continue to cause excruciating pain and immobility.

However, being a thoughtful and well-read man, Norman Cousins began to think deeply concerning his situation. First, he wondered why it was that he should have this disease. He remembered that prior to and during his initial symptoms, he had been enduring a situation of great distress. A large factor within this distressing situation was his own sense of powerlessness to change the problem and his profound discouragement as a result. As described in the journal *Science*, researchers at Harvard Medical School have shown that rats who undergo similar stressors over which they have no control do show signs of biochemical changes that indicate vulnerability to disease.

Mr. Cousins wondered whether this internal environment of discouragement was a key factor in allowing a disease process to begin and gain strength against his life. He also was aware of growing evidence that the strength of immunity and personal belief are closely tied together. This research is well reviewed in an article entitled "Training the Mind to Heal," by Lois Wingerson.

In a new sub-specialty, psychoneuroimmunology, Robert Ader, a psychiatry professor at the University of Rochester, New York, has developed data showing that the brain's information flows almost instantly to the immune system, which then affects hormonal balance, and the subsequent creation, release, and action of many kinds of life-sustaining systems. Belief is brain information, as we already know, affecting the bio-electrical stream toward health.

Norman Cousins knew he had been discouraged. At times he had perceived his situation to be beyond his own help to change it; he had begun to believe deeply in this negative perception. If these negative beliefs contributed to his disease, would a change of perception about his condition and a positive belief in his own will to live, help to change his own disease process into health again?

Mr. Cousins felt this question was worth his own experimental and conscious effort to seek an answer. Requesting the assistance of his physician, Norman Cousins developed a plan that would strengthen his chances of recovery. Although his doctor did not himself agree with every detail of the plan, he knew that his patient's only chance to live was involved in a personal commitment and strength of will.

Mr. Cousins details his plan in his own book,

Happiness And Healing

which is well worth a thoughtful reading. Many factors within this plan lead to an eventual healing and life change. We will review those aspects of the Cousins plan that coincide with the threads of Endorphin ideas we have explored.

In an effort to strengthen a positive attitude, Norman Cousins decided to try the conscious use of laughter. He read joke books, watched Candid Camera clips, and countless comedies on movie film. In a conscious change of perception, Mr. Cousins encouraged himself to laugh with great energy at all the gags within these films, even the silliest and most stupid. And, he didn't settle for smiling or snickering at the comic situations. He chose to allow himself to laugh so heavily that his entire body laughed with him. To his surprise and delight, Mr. Cousins found that there was an anesthetic effect from ten minutes of deep laughter. This therpeutic effect then lasted two hours—allowing him pain-free sleep. When the pain returned, he then played his comedies, often to be relieved from pain once again.

Indeed, this pain-free sleep had not been achieved previously, even by high and frequent doses of Demerol, the strong narcotic opiate his doctor had prescribed for pain. Pain relief equal to or better than Demerol? This is our Endorphin clue. Could laughter actually release the natural, pain-relieving biochemistry which Demerol mimics?

❋ ❋ ❋

Laughter and Positive Emotions

One of the pain-killing therapies used in today's clinics and hospitals is nitrous oxide or "laughing gas." A new application of this treatment has been tried on terminally ill cancer patients. The results give us a better understanding of why laughing gas works. Nitrous oxide freed one patient from pain for "the first time in months" according to a July, 1983, article from United Press International.

While decreasing pain, anxiety, and agitation, the use of nitrous oxide also improves appetite, mood, and the capacity to communicate with others. These clues indicate that nitrous oxide, through some laughter mechanism, could well be an Endorphin trigger. The connection between Endorphins and laughter has been suggested by Dr. Avram Goldstein of Stanford University. (He was the researcher who conceived of the lock and keyhole actions of opiates and Endorphins.)

In the book *Laugh After Laugh*, Dr. Raymond A. Moody discusses the potential which laughter and humor have for healing. He cites many examples of a humorous approach as being useful for decrease in pain, a way out of depression and withdrawal, and as an assistant method for the reinforcement of inherent healing mechanisms.

It is interesting to note that much of Dr. Moody's writing, developed prior to Endorphin discoveries, would point to research that would soon confirm a physiological, biochemical mechanism for the findings he cited. The descriptions of the improved quality of experience are yet another indication that some biochemicals, or combinations of them—which include Endorphins—are induced by laughter, and are a powerful potential for the biochemistry that gives us a sense of well-being and quality.

Dr. Moody makes the important, recurring observation that health and the regaining of health after illness are facilitated by a special kind of attitude. This view looks at the world with a sense of humor about oneself and one's surroundings. The chance of regaining health is improved when an ill person can take a comic perspective about life, while yet retaining a positive, loving, and respectful view of himself and others.

This description of an attitude implies a balanced biochemistry, a balanced perspective of one's own condition, and the people and events that affect this condition. Such an attitude implies high levels of Endorphins, which assist with a "comic sense" or euphoria, also linked with immune strength and healing.

Through the comic perspective that laughter provided, Norman Cousins began to increase his positive belief about his own life. Gradually then, through months of strengthening exercise, improved diet, and continuing laughter, Mr. Cousins applied his renewed faith to the physical demands of health. Of course, he did become free of the constraint of disease.

155

Norman Cousins still lives, healthy and active, beyond the grim prognosis of imminent and painful death.

Galen Clark simply decided to interact within a beautiful environment before dying. Norman Cousins took up a conscious, therapeutic plan to change his internal perception about his environment. Both stories increase our understanding of the definition of enrichment. Both stories tell of men courageous enough to interact with a distressful situation and thus transform that situation into eustress.

Probing Negativity

Both stories hint at the important role of positive belief, which searches for happiness despite and beyond the seeming solitary cage of distress and extreme illness. Consider the irony that while we search for external assistance, the biochemical potential for pleasure and happiness exists within the reality of Endorphins, and that this potential for euphoria and pain-freedom streams through our biochemical design. Why aren't we always happy? When we are troubled and unhappy, why is that so? Might this condition reflect a biochemical imbalance that can somehow be corrected within the bioelectrical stream of consciousness? A negative consciousness, attitude, or perception might indeed hinder health or block the flow of health-sustaining biochemicals, such as Endorphins.

How is it that we could then move through or around the seeming perceptual blockages in the stream of consciousness that seem to underlie the feelings of distress and a subsequent flow toward disease?

To answer this question, let's think about how we begin our experience in life and how we begin our responses to, our opinions about, that experience. We develop habits, attitudes, and perceptions of response to an environment that seems, at that time, to stand still. This is especially true when the environment is perceived to be uncomfortable, discouraging, or threatening. During that time of distress, we come to develop a response which may well be the most appropriate or useful at that time. But then this bio-chemical habit becomes etched into the bio-electrical process of our being.

Life changes again, the threatening experience does not remain fixed within our environment, but the response does. In this way, we come to believe that our perception of life holds the only true reality of our world. And yet, all around us, others develop different responses to, and perceptions about, this same flow or experience. The stream continues on, yet we, who are still bogged down by the blockage of our own response to that threatening event back there, around a bend in the past, do not perceive the present stream and its true potential. We can become so entrenched in yesterday's negative bio-electrical responses that we become unable to perceive today's true reality. Our response to that which seems to threaten us solidifies our perception of life and may begin to stunt the growth and branching of brain dendrites and to stagnate the stream of brain potential.

Risking The Heights of Growth

Another example about remission and healing illustrates the story of a man named Herbert Howe who developed a way to overcome the dread disease of terminal bone cancer and his own sense of distress about this disease.

In his autobiography called, *Do Not Go Gentle*, Herbert Howe describes yet another interactive plan to enrich a distressed and diseased environment. Herbert Howe was an athlete, active in running and soccer. He had developed a small lump on his wrist that began to give him pain. When a biopsy was taken, both he and his physician were amazed and concerned to learn that his lump was malignant. Indeed, he had a cancer so rare that it had been recorded in medical history less than one hundred times. This situation seemed very grim for Herbert Howe. With this kind of cancer producing a high percentage of fatality within five years, the diagnosis was devastating. But, Herbert Howe was a young man, still in graduate school, wishing for enough time to finish his thesis, find a good job, marry and raise a family.

Again, like both Clark and Cousins, Herbert Howe began to consider what he could do about his condition. He desired to interact individually with the disease-and-distress processes in his life. He had always been an active, athletic person. When it was suggested by his friends that he try to maintain his active hobbies, he thought to himself that while sports are not a cure for cancer, his life remaining would be pleasanter for him. Thus, he pursued an increasing, vigorous routine of touch football, running, squash, and swimming.

In addition to Herbert's choice to continue athletics actively, he opted to follow the therapeutic plans of his doctors. This meant that, as the story continued for the next year, he endured the painful side effects of radiation and chemotherapy treatments.

As the title of his book implies, Herbert Howe did not spoil himself or give in to the immense discomfort and distress he felt during this time. He simply focused upon leading a life additional to the life of a cancer patient. Despite extreme nausea and weakness, he ran and swam whenever he could. As a result, he found that he felt better, not only physically, but also emotionally and mentally. As long as he could, he maintained his graduate school work and tutorial assignments.

He tells of how he would become overwhelmingly discouraged by being so ill and not being able to control his distress response to those symptoms. But, as the weeks went on, he continued to maintain his vigorous exercise schedule whenever possible. Although he could not always master his feelings of total discouragement, he never gave up, believing that, for himself, fighters had a better chance to win.

One day, Herbert began to wonder whether his exercise program actually could be reducing his sense of distress over his physical situation. As he was developing his own plan to improve his response to stress, scientists in Rome were working with studies showing that physical exercise releases both Beta-Endorphin and ACTH, the hormones now known to work together in building health.

As described in the European journal *Experimentia*, this study, which used human subjects rather than laboratory rats, showed that large increases in both hormones were especially noted with maximal physical effort. The authors of this experiment were careful to leave physiological speculation about these findings for others to consider. But, as we continue with Herbert Howe's story, we can use his example to consider the significance of this data about exercise, ACTH, Endorphins, and the regaining of health.

When, because of his treatment regimen, Herbert was unable to complete the doctoral thesis he had cherished so much, he decided that he needed something else to confirm his belief in his own innate ability too overcome obstacles. Remembering the achievement he had felt when completing a challenging canoe race, he began an even more vigorous training program to prepare again for that same upcoming competition.

While describing these months of extreme physical hardship, Herbert Howe discusses his gradual changes of perception about himself, his achievements, his ability to adapt to the seemingly negative changes in his life, and his beliefs about life's meaning. In his youth, Howe saw sports from the perspective of defeating the competition. But, through illness, his idea about sports changed into battles against the challenges of chemotherapy and his own negative responses to the situation. As in preparing for athletic achievement, Howe sustained himself through these trials with definite goals for improving strength and stamina.

While training for the upcoming marathon he planned to enter with a companion athlete, Howe and his friend prepared physically and psychologically for the endurance. From the first, they knew that there would be no way in which they could even begin to come close to winning. Their canoe was old and heavy—no match for the sleeker, lighter canoes the professionals were using. But, their goal and perception about their possibilities were defined differently. That difference was the concept which gave their plan meaning. They would complete the race despite the handicap of cancer, and exceed their own previous accomplishment in time, giving this race the best they could give, physically as well as emotionally and mentally.

On the day of the race, they were able to surpass their own goals. Twelve arduous hours after the two young men had begun the race, the spectators who helped them at the finish line observed that they had truly won the unofficial division of "clunkers." Indeed, Herbert and his teammate had completed the canoe race two hours faster than their previous time. And, they had exceeded their expectations for themselves by a significant margin, completing the course one hour sooner than they had hoped.

Herbert Howe likened this canoeing experience to

his change in perception about his own ability to respond to the distress of disease and chemotherapy. He outlived the dire predictions given with his diagnosis. But, most importantly, he felt that he had a new belief about himself and his growing capacities.

Herbert Howe went on to graduate and achieve his doctorate from Harvard and work as an international journalist.

From this example, we do not necessarily suggest that everyone take up the kind of marathon approach to disease and distress which Herbert Howe used. Mr. Howe's positive belief system was entwined with his ability to be a super-achieving athlete. At the conclusion of his story, Herbert speculates on how his own healing experience through sports might be applied to many differing perceptions, attitudes, and lifestyles. Other activities, such as crafts, artistic and musical endeavors, or gardening, could help someone through the painful and humiliating times of illness.

At the close of his book, Mr. Howe mentions the Simonton work we reviewed in Chapter Three. He discusses the Simontons' key observations about those flexible patients who seek out changes in their own perception about distress and disease. These patients are less likely to blame others for their troubles and feel less despondent, becoming increasingly self-sufficient and self-accepting.

Mr. Howe's story is a dramatic example of how the physical body's condition of disease can be changed through deliberate choices to maintain a positive belief about oneself and to apply that on-ing attitude to a plan that includes involving all aspects of oneself—body, mind, emotions, and spirit.

We have reviewed three stories about healing and increasing happiness. Three men, Clark, Cousins, and Howe, of different times, ideas, and plans, were able to continue their lives, become happier, and grow beyond their sense of distress and imprisonment within disease. They developed new perceptions about themselves and their situations. And the biochemical flow of their brains was somehow changed, perhaps through these efforts, to support health rather than disease, happiness rather than hopelessness and despair.

Herbert Howe's story is an example of a man who may have learned to trigger Endorphins. He found, as he went along with his experiment to change his life, that his body reinforced his choices and began to respond with invigorated health.

In an article for the journal *Perspectives in Biology and Medicine*, Dr. Daniel Carr proposes that Endorphins somehow reinforce "goal-directed behavior." This concept is exemplified in Herbert Howe's victory. Is it possible that through this kind of biochemical mechanism, Endorphins reinforce our health? We can certainly see how Endorphins might reinforce the kinds of behavior we are told will keep us healthy, like regular exercise, intake of adequate nourishment, and proper sleep habits, as well as reinforce our ability to cope with stress.

However, as we know, Endorphins can also, through past bonding, reinforce behavior which would be destructive to our health.

This idea is also described in a recent article written for the self-help journal, *Rx Being Well*. Dr. James P. Carter explains that Endorphins may well be one of the biochemical reinforcements of unhealthy habits. When we find ourselves addicted to learned compulsions, such as the use of nicotine or alcohol, driving fast or recklessly, staying awake too long or preferring a sedentary lifestyle, Endorphins play a role in the reinforcement of, or bonding to, unhealthy choices. In this case, electrical biochemistry can signal the undoing of our health through its imperative to unwise choices of behavior.

Welcoming Change

Consider that an enriched, health and life-sustaining environment includes a welcoming perspective concerning change. We know that change is a stimulus that triggers an Endorphin response. We seek out change for the joy of it. We love to shop for new things like cars, motorcycles, and boats. In our homes, we love to remodel kitchens or hang new wallpaper. We look for new vacation spots or restaurants we haven't tried before. We find a sense of freshness in these endeavors and even feel good while planning changes as we thumb through catalogues or travel books. But, is this anticipation for change always a beneficial and euphoric response?

An answer to that question might depend upon our own individual perception of change. As mentioned earlier, the enriched rats were not preconditioned to perceive their changing environment as a threat.   They simply interacted with their new toys and thus seemed to benefit from doing so.

But our lives are more complex. We have learned to love, to bond, to find happiness in certain places, people, things, and habits of being.   A change which means the loss of that which is dear to us or that which we cling to might not seem to be a beneficial change. This kind of loss through change might appear threatening and create a malignant rather than an enriching environment. As we have explored before, a change may be interpreted, by our unconscious limbic and reptilian brain biochemistry, as a signal of rejection or defeat.   Thus, this loss may begin a corresponding biochemical breakdown of immune defenses; a biochemical perception which opens the door for disease processes like major infections, and even cancer, to enter.

Or, our bodies can biochemically over-compensate for change and loss by building an overactive immune defense. As we have reviewed in Chapter Three, arthritis has been linked to a hyperactive biochemical response.

In scientific data which study human response to change, significant findings have shown that any overload of changes in life situations can be stressful enough to trigger life-threatening disease processes. Yet, these major life changes need not be sad ones, involving loss; changes that threaten health can be seemingly happy ones, such as job promotions or buying a home.   The key ingredient in these studies about change is the concept of overload. One good change might be invigorating.   One bad change might be reasonably tolerable. But several changes stacked together—good and/or bad—or one major change, such as the loss of a spouse, might be enough to cause the major distress leading to disease.

You may have noticed that a couple, long and happily married, often die within a close time period of each other. Common sense tells us that grief has killed the surviving one. Now scientific discovery about brain biochemistry enhances this common observation. Endorphins are somehow involved in the bonding, loving process. A loss of love or a perceived loss of love might be the distressful overload which would signal an Endorphin imbalance and begin an immunity shutdown leading to life-threatening illness and death.

We know that, through the action of our powerful Endorphins, biochemical loss of any kind can cause perceived pain and distress. Through the euphoric bonding and loving of a happy marriage, one could become biochemically addicted to the presence of a spouse. We might find ourselves addicted to those conditions which make us happy—addicted to our own sense of being loved. But this loving is not just emotional or just psychological. This loving is a perception involving physiology, a bio-electrical and biochemical bonding. It is the euphoria we feel during pleasurable moments with the ones beloved to us, or when we experience a great oneness with life, itself.

We are often comforted by a seeming constancy of life. We glean security from a rhythm which reflects this perception. But then, as we know, life continues on, and inevitable changes come, large and small, shocking or beneficial, but adding up to stress that brings possible distress, not just emotionally or from a purely psychological origin, but, again, from a biochemical physiology where disease and threats to life begin. Instead of worrying however that the changing moments, days, and years somehow threaten us with calamity or unknown trouble, we can consider that the changing moments really represent the flow of life's ongoing stimulus toward growth and the euphoric eustress of becoming.

It may be that we anticipate the future as containing something we'd like to prevent. We may even try to control this potentially negative outcome, guarding against the possibility of impending loss. But we will be preparing effectively for that future moment only if our present awareness contains receptive responses that are unhindered by a constant review of the past or worry about the future.

A focus upon the past or future can become a slip in perception that biochemically distorts present reality. If we continually perceive a past loss or prepare against a future loss, in reality we lose today's interactive potential for becoming.

Dr. Neil Fiore, the stress-management psychologist we met in previous chapters, has explained that our best and only true coping mechanism is the perception that our bodies and beings have the capacity to meet effectively whatever ongoing changes may occur. He reminds us that we are designed that way.

Review of Endorphin findings helps to underline these realizations. Powerful brain biochemicals, waiting to meet the stress of changes, good and bad, help us to live effectively within the present, on-going patterns of challenge and joy.

When we are depressed or feel impossibly locked into one way of being, we wonder how we might make a change within ourselves and flow into another way of being. Sometimes we feel so entrenched that we endure the vicious cycles of repetitive experiences which can imprison us in unwelcome ruts for years and even for a lifetime. These well-worn trenches, however, might not be the dead-end mazes they seem to be.

An example of this idea has been developed by Richard Kimball, a social psychologist who uses the stress of risk and a corresponding response to change as a dramatic therapy. In New Mexico, at the Santa Fe Mountain Center for criminal rehabilitation, Dr. Kimball assists clients, who are deviants—among them, murderers, rapists, child molesters, armed robbers, former drug addicts, prostitutes, and juvenile delinquents. Within Kimball's therapeutic plan, he confronts his clients with the awesome need of risking their lives on dangerous mountain-climbing expeditions. Through this process, men and women who have previously limited their own happiness to the harm of others, or of themselves, have a chance to stretch to a new becoming.

In an interview for the magazine *People*, Kimball explains that this imposed risk potentially produces a growth that would not occur if his clients were comfortable and unafraid.

Our own Endorphin explorations are reflected in

the thoughts of one man who made discoveries about his life during a winter ascent of a rugged mountain. Through this experience, he no longer saw himself as just a child molester; but as someone who could face his problems with a sense of self-worth.

Perhaps this man found a new way to induce Endorphins through the stress response. He was able to reverse previously learned criminal behavior to become "high" from a positive, successful, achievement experience that criminals don't often have a chance to have.

We are not locked in to one behavior or one balance of biochemistry that supports that behavior by euphorically reinforcing its action. In this case, physical, mental, and emotional risk toward growth changed a physical behavior which had been supported by mental and emotional deviancy. An Endorphin stress response to change may have assisted the process from distressed being to growth and becoming.

A Resolution of Conflict

We may have come to know ourselves as fixed beings, already molded by people and events, now set like a statue in marble or concrete and standing unmoved by the subtle flow of change. Or we may feel ourselves to be in a rut which seems to grow narrower or deeper, enclosing life's experience with boredom and lack of possibilities. Thus, we may long for the tide of change to wash over us and transform our dull lives.

How is it that an ongoing flow of biochemicals, such as Endorphins, with infinite potential for the enriching experiences of life, could reflect the seeming prisons in which we find ourselves?

Remember back to Chapter One and Karl Pribram's holographic brain theory. Our brains harbor multi-sensory images which are maintained through our own individual bio-electricity. Our brains' sense of reality is shaped and reshaped by these multi-sensory images and their potential to be transformed. Within this concept, the products of our mind—thoughts, perceptions, attitudes, feelings, reactions, opinions and judgments—color our sense of reality, the environment we find ourselves in, and our own responses to this individual reality.

From this concept, we can modify our definition of the word *stress*. Stress is a reality which our muti-sensory imagery might perceive. Within this perception, we have a feeling of challenge, perhaps of risk or conflict. Stress can be considered as the perceived environment wherein, through the brain's imagery, conflict or conflict potential is sensed.

Within this interpretation of stress as conflict imagery, distress may be defined as these same images locked in conflict. Somehow, the sense or feeling of being imprisoned defines the sense of distress, as though there seems no way out from the confronting challenge. This imagery of imprisonment may reflect previously learned inadequacy or limitation. Or, it may seem that all known doors out have been tried, and there appears to be no escape from the perceived conflict of bio-electrical images within the brain.

This sense of distressed imagery may indeed be one of the beginning messages which our brains encode before a disease process begins. This distress brain imagery may be the biochemical code which calls the immune response into action, over-reaction, or even lack of action. As we have explored before, both over-active and under-active immune responses can lead to illness by disrupting the balanced maintenance of health. In disease, our bodies, like the distress of our brain's imagery, are imprisoned in a condition which may seem beyond escaping. Being ill seems being stagnated—cut off from the flow of becoming well.

But, as Hans Selye has reminded us, there is yet another kind of stress. This stress, which is exhilarating and euphoric, finds a potential or real resolution to the conflict-distress imagery. Somehow, a self-imposed restriction within the prison of conflict is re-routed to flow again in an imagery of freedom— the condition called eustress that seems to be supported by the bio-electricity of euphoric Endorphins. Norman Cousins laughed. Galen Clark interacted with the beauty of nature. Herbert Howe drove his physical body to maximum effort. A criminal risked his life upon a snowy mountainside. All found a way to risk the heights of growth and resolve their conflicts. All were able to kindle the flame of a health-giving bio-electrical fire within their lives. Perhaps, in all of these cases, Endorphins flowed with fresh abundance to reinforce new choices and restore health, both physically and psychologically.

Risk-takers elicit their stress-Endorphin response by laying their physical lives on the line. The risk toward physical, emotional, mental, and even spiritual growth is a similar stimulus, but less life-threatening. The perception of threat is often there, stopping many for perhaps years or a lifetime from risking a change of being. But we, who are learning about the induction of euphoric biochemical happenings through the presence of Endorphins, might feel inclined to take the risk toward growth within a challenging situation. We might be more willing to seek new answers, like Norman Cousins, or to develop our potential, like Herbert Howe. We might risk the chance of seeking enrichment within the seeming cage of our lives. Like Galen Clark, we might decide to take a leap in consciousness; to say Yes with Dr. Prigogine to the potential chaos of change within and trust the outcome to be a fuller transformation. Nature teaches us this perspective. A tree stands, awaiting the seasons to decide the course of its growth. We are also a product of nature's evolutionary process; we are uniquely designed for choice. We can choose how the changing seasons and life's cycles will affect us.

***

Diversifying Joy

Remember the laboratory cage, a prison for solitary animals who became enriched by the experimental design of a changing environment. In this same way, the cage of distress may be enriched by images of change or newness which can then flow to begin the eustress process.

But what images may we give ourselves that will effect a perception—or attitude-change within our brain's biochemistry?

We may physically receive a new flow of enrichment and eustress by our perceived appreciation of an enhanced, five-sensory awareness. Our five senses may well be vital stimulus avenues, triggering our ongoing euphoria.

Melvin Konner, a biological anthropologist at Harvard University, relates a story of the power of sensory appreciation in his book, *The Tangled Wing, Biological Constraints on the Human Spirit*. A male chimpanzee was studied in a national park in Tanzania. Here, the chimp had been followed to a spectacular waterfall which cascaded twenty-five feet, to spray a rainbow mist into the surrounding tropical forest. At the water's edge, the chimpanzee waited for no apparent reason except, perhaps, to contemplate.

He then became excited, calling out in a hooting sound, running around and pounding trees with his fists. He seemed compelled to some sort of ecstatic action at the beautiful sight, for there was no other apparent reason for this behavior. Day after day, he repeated his journey to the waterfall, his contemplation, and his joyous calling. Then, other chimpanzees journeyed to the waterfall as well. They had plenty of water elsewhere to drink. They didn't need to cross the lake to another vicinity. It seemed they simply wondered at the beauty of the scene they perceived, and felt compelled to joy—perhaps by their own reverberating bio-electricity—to dance and sing.

What sensory images do you experience that bring joy and give meaning to your life? The vision of sunlight gilds the world to an image far more precious than a safe filled with gold coins. Color, texture, and pattern offer us infinite potential and variety to behold and enjoy. The ongoing awareness of beauty which you can receive may be a potent Endorphin trigger toward the happiness in your life. The imagery vision of a beautiful world is an appreciative perception which can ease your sense of distress and increase your sense of eustress.

Give yourself the potential Endorphin trigger of appreciating sensory awareness. Any fragrance that you love can reach into the deepest recesses of your instinctual brain to bless your day, while diminishing its cares. Piney woods, fresh-mown grass, the sting of ocean spray, even one fragrant flower—what are your favorite aromas? Seek them out and discover new ones.

Remember how important your sense of taste can be to the quality of life. Take your meals more slowly and relish the tastes you have chosen. Try new flavors and change your recipes. If you are heavier than you'd like to be, perhaps you've used taste as an

Endorphin trigger too often or too consistently. You may not realize that an invigorating walk or new hobby may provide the kind of biochemical high a chocolate bar can trigger. And these new ways of feeling good will increase your metabolism and help you burn calories.

If you have a strong tactile sense, perhaps touch sensations can bring you joy. Silky, smooth, and rough are all potential textures to enliven your awareness. If you have never noticed the thrill of tactile sensations before, give yourself to some exploration. A small touch may surprise you with a sense of unsuspected pleasure. Warmth, chill, and massage are all known sensory and therapeutic tools for the relief of tension and pain. These sensations, electrical and biochemical messages, can help to ease your sense of distress or heighten a moment's awareness.

Sound, too, can be a precious instrument of happiness. How many beautiful tones do we miss by lack of attention? Breezes whisper and leaves rustle. Brooks rush or tinkle or glide. Tides roar. Snow falls in eloquent silence. Laughter, both experienced and heard, is a known biochemical flow of joy. A bird bursts into song, bringing melody into the world.

Do birds derive joy from the music they share? In an intriguing study recorded in an issue of the journal *Brain Research*, Dr. Susan M. Ryan and her colleagues have found that there is a high level of Endorphin-related activity in the vocal cords of a finch.

Have you ever experienced a chill up and down

your spine while listening to music? Do you wonder about the pleasure and relaxation music can provide you? Dr. Avram Goldstein, the Endorphin researcher who connected laughter with Endorphins, also wondered about music and completed a study showing that the spine-chill response to music indicates high Endorphins in your body.

This tingling experience is a bio-electrical happening which cascades down the spinal cord to swiftly disappear, becoming the briefest moment of sensation in time. As we have learned, this flow of energy has a profound effect on our well-being, even after the cascade has passed.

But, have you ever noticed that when you try to think logically about this chill you have had, it disappears as though you have thought it away? Perhaps there is a cortical, intellectual shut-off valve blocking the flow of this response which contributes to relaxation and well-being.

This finding gives us yet another clue about the feeling of well-being, probably assisted by Endorphins. We know that a large number of Endorphin keyholes are found within our own emotional limbic brain. The physiological place that feels pleasure and pain responds to musical vibration from listening ears, or receives beautiful smells and delicious tastes.

An ongoing pleasure in life, that can ease our distress and increase our eustress, requires an interactive approach to living. Although we might prefer to watch television or to sit on a park bench while the world goes by, these activities do less for the changes in our bio-electrical flow. Remember the solitary laboratory rat whose neighbors played with toys. Watching the experience of someone else does not trigger the same biochemical response that our own explorations can have for our brains. Dendrites branch and grow in response to our own interactions with, and explorations of, life.

Give yourself the Endorphin trigger of increased and interesting activity. If you are not athletic or your body has lost its conditioning, begin today. You needn't walk far or fast to experience the euphoric biochemical high that a jogger might require hours to feel.

If you are athletic, you may have noticed that you've come to depend upon a lengthy regimen to feel good. Or, your biochemical tolerance to activity may now give you a sense of boredom. Try a new activity—play volleyball on the beach, go dancing or swimming, or backpack a forested trail. Risk a new interactive hobby, such as exploring white water rapids. Change your physical activity and you will broaden your base for a biochemical high.

And, if you are chronically handicapped or ill and your range of experience is limited in some way, you have all the more reason to seek out the kinds of Endorphin triggers that may be available to you. Find a way to broaden your awareness and your experience. You especially need high doses of biochemical joy in order to maximize your health and happiness.

If you are cutting down on, or trying to quit, smoking, drinking, or other habits that are potentially harmful to your life, consider that you can find alternative forms of pleasure. Endorphins are not just created by external substances. Remember that external substances, from heroin to food, give pleasure because an internal biochemical mechanism and its potential always exist, awaiting internal triggering.

Change is a stressor which can be triggered for enrichment, but too much change can quickly become distressful. When your life requires major changes, good or otherwise, you can assist yourself with these changes by triggering your euphoric biochemistry; broaden your base of happiness, search for joy wherever you can find it, and appreciate the simple pleasures available to you. Remember how invigorating change can be. Use simple changes if you like; drive a different route to work or brew a new kind of tea.

When catastrophic change occurs in your life, you may notice a desire for extra rest or withdrawal from the seeming tidal wave overwhelming you. At these times, renewal becomes your need. Then, restful input, such as music, reading, or a reflective, inspirational focus, can become a *recharging* stimulus toward the ongoing flow of your brain's biochemistry.

Other Endorphin triggers might include completing a project or plan about which you have been procrastinating. You might trigger biochemical eustress by applying yourself to a challenge you have been resisting, or learning a subject or skill you never thought you could master. All of these ideas are examples of a positive interaction with the stress of euphoric change.

As we grow older, we are particularly prone to limit our enrichment to ways of being or of conditions in the past, when we were younger. Or we might again experience life's growth, vicariously, through the youth of our children or grandchildren. Dendrite growth within the brain is not limited by age, but becomes stunted by inactivity. Most of us can think of examples of older folk who remain vibrant, leading quality lives as octogenarians and beyond. In some way, they have tapped into the ongoing life force, from "being to becoming," maintaining a freshness of attitude and belief.

Perhaps it would be useful to you to consider your own friends who have thus succeeded. What have you learned about Endorphins that apply to these examples—their lifestyle, their choices, their ability to cope with trouble and their focus upon life's joys? Just because we are past our youth, (or first youth) we needn't deny ourselves a child's fresh perspective and interaction with life. The biblical suggestion to "be as little children" is often cited as good advice.

This also applies to our Endorphin exploration. We still can be awed by the beauty of a rainbow. None of us is too old to blow soap bubbles. Perhaps we would like to sail a toy boat in a pond or take a rubber duck to our bath or jacuzzi. Maybe we'd like a railroad set for Christmas or to play with dolls again. If something innovative interests us, like a computer or video game, there is no good reason for not trying to recapture a sense of youthful potential by learning about it. We need to release the feeling of inadequacy, age, or lack of skill. We could take up bird-watching or experiment with the harmonica. We can always discover ways and reasons to find our own bio-electrical reverberation, to laugh and play and sing.

As stress is an Endorphin trigger, perhaps this same biochemical process has helped you bond to a difficult, distasteful, or terrible situation in the past. Bad memories may seem so etched in your brain that you may feel forced to relive guilt or anger, resentment or bitterness, over and over again. But, as we have come to learn, this is brain imagery that is biochemical. The brain's physiology does not differentiate between a present challenging situation and a distressed image recalled from the past. It simply responds with biochemical actions to prepare the body for that distress.

Thus, we can stress and distress ourselves far too long and hard over a past situation. Perhaps this is why forgiveness comes so highly recommended from counselors of many faiths and beliefs. Forgiveness is a freeing imagery, giving over to the inevitable changes of life. Forgiveness may be one of the attitudes which biochemically releases the brain to seek new enrichment. It may allow new dendrites to grow and new bio-electrical synapses to be ignited. Perhaps forgiveness is even an Endorphin trigger.

The Key Within

One of the most thought-provoking areas within our Endorphin exploration brings us to the age-old question that may seem more philosophical than scientific. How is life's quality defined? In today's world, many of us find ourselves exclusively pursuing the goods of the material world to supply our sense of life's quality. We seek after nice things, beautiful possessions. We seek after having a good time, meeting someone and having that person fall in love with us. We seek after having beautiful, talented, well-behaved children. We are socialized to believe that things or events happening to us within our environment are the reasons for our happiness or unhappiness. And, if we miss out on that which we desire, we believe that we will be missing out on life and life's quality, missing out on the rewards of our pursuit of happiness.

But, Endorphin ideas have helped us to explore the concept that happiness potential is inherent within. When we are happy and euphoric, biochemistry supports this resonating feeling. We can recall stories of poor people who are happy. Many who look back realize that their parents were very poor but also very happy and seemingly rich because of a special quality in their lives. These fortunate ones have the quality of sharing, caring, and loving each other, a quality of family, a flexibility of attitude, optimism, and enthusiasm for life and its potential. We also hear of individuals with massive amounts of capital, perhaps with beautiful homes, with planes and boats. Often, these same people seem beset with problems, challenges that rob them of their happiness. They may wish to simplify, to unburden themselves; they wonder sometimes if they would have to be poor to become happy again.

Happiness can be defined as a quality of resonance that reverberates within our own bio-electrical systems, a special biochemical balance, a stream maintaining a flow from being to becoming. This same flow could stagnate should we linger too long in the past or the future. That is not to say that we, who live in the Western World, should give up our striving, all sense of progress, all sense of desire or wishing for achievement, possessions, or happiness in relationships with others. But, the forced, unrelenting striving after that which could lock us biochemically into a sense of bondage to this striving and to our desires—this is a sense of distress which ultimately could rob us of our health and make that elusive happiness even harder to discover.

The exploration of Endorphin discoveries helps to give a new meaning to the terms happiness and quality. What does it mean to be healthy, wealthy, and wise? Is it possible that our biochemistry is designed to resonate toward these goals? Is a happy life assisted by the capability to fine-tune receptive awareness toward appreciation and the ongoing kindling of a biochemical euphoric response?

When we succeed outwardly and know prosperity when we have larger paychecks or better homes or prettier children or more loving spouses or more exciting trips and adventures—even when we achieve these desires, if we haven't developed a way to trigger and maintain an internal euphoric response to these environments, these same desires will someday seem stale. Thus, we will always be wanting for something or someone else. The grass will still be greener on the other side of the fence. It could be said that, physiologically and psychologically, our wealth lies within our own euphoric, bio-electrical responses to life. As in the wise investment of material riches, wealth is stronger, broader, and more stable if it is diversified and invested in a wide range of interests and activities, instead of placed into one venture or bank account—or source of happiness.

Dr. James A. Knight, who is a professor of Psychiatry at Louisiana State School of Medicine and also an ordained minister, has explained that true happiness is a kind of spiritual homeostasis or "will to meaning." Through this process, we find ourselves reverberating to that purpose in life that is uniquely ours to live. If we can find that mission or direction in life, we can sustain that ongoing sense of renewal which we seek in the qualities of health and happiness. Dr. Knight reminds us never to underestimate the capacity of both mind and body to be renewed and regenerated.

Endorphin research adds a new dimension to this concept. Like Clark, Cousins, and Howe, we can flow through or around the seeming distress barriers of life. Dr. Knight suggests that this process is one of converting negative force into positive power by appreciating, even cherishing, our own natural drives to find that balance resonating within ourselves.

It is interesting to note that Dr. Knight would use the electrical concept of converting negative power to positive. Endorphins are biochemicals of our own body's electricity. Through this discovery, we can better understand how Dr. Knight's psychological and spiritual advice can be supported physiologically by the electrical biochemistry of euphoria.

Take another look back down life's stream that is your past. What did those golden moments have in common? Perhaps you felt love or gave love or shared a rich sense of belonging. A moment of earthly beauty seemed to have the sheen of heaven upon it. It may have been a long-awaited time such as a wedding day or a special vacation; or a simple time, the warmth of a sunbath, the crisp chill of autumn air. Perhaps a birdsong lifted an afternoon for you or an orchard's fragrance wafted across the hills to you. Maybe rain sang upon a roof. Fire crackled to set a hearth aglow in the evening darkness. Stars pierced a desert sky; snow peaks etched a horizon. A child's hug warmed your heart. You remember a job well done, a mountain climbed.

A heightened sensory awareness bonds with profound meaning and the worshipping and loving of life. An extraordinary biochemical balance reverberates to brighten the mind, nourish the body, and replenish the soul, even now, with golden awareness.

These moments string across our days and tempt us to feel that we no longer can have what is gone forever. But these moments are truly our wealth if we use our past experience to heighten our appreciation of present beauty.

Or, do you find yourself tempted to look up the stream into your immediate future—to tonight's candlelight dinner or the upcoming "Michelobe" weekend. Perhaps your vacation comes soon, or a promotion next year.

When tried by relationships, we tend to wish, for example, that our children were through this terrible phase or that a difficult family member would just go away. We hear ourselves saying, "I wish I were in love again." Maybe, even on that long-awaited vacation, we think about when our plane will land or the view of a quaint town around the bend. We get so caught up in the biochemical process of wishing, anticipating, clock-watching, waiting for the next coffee break or early retirement, that again, the all-important present moment and its beautiful potential slips away to be an unknown pebble in the stream of time.

Is it possible that when we feel fully alive, a vibrancy of brain biochemicals resonates this feeling in the present moment? Such questions arise again, waiting for experience and exploration to answer, continuing the process that flows from being to becoming. Like hopes and dreams, questions point us toward further search and growth. Dendrites stretch, branching beyond previous experience and limitation to seek further enrichment and awareness. Powerful euphoric Endorphins, natural biochemicals of pleasure, eustress, joy, even ecstacy and health, flow with the potential to carry radiance to any given moment of a day. Somehow a special bio-electrical balance can be quickened. Somehow an Endorphin response begins to reverberate the euphoria of living.

Endorphins may indeed be triggered through positive expectancy, through capturing the glistening present moment with receptive awareness, through the focus of appreciation and cherishing. That spark of euphoria may also be found in the releasement of all which could imprison or distress.

Let us throw out the moldy images of resentment and guilt. Dusty, stale, nostalgic bittersweets cannot compare with today's freshness. Perhaps tomorrow's experience will be finer than today's. But today's receptive focusing upon present joys can help to sharpen tomorrow's skill in appreciating the world we will find then. Tomorrow's fulfilled being will reflect today's ongoing ecstatic becoming—the gift of our Endorphin connection.

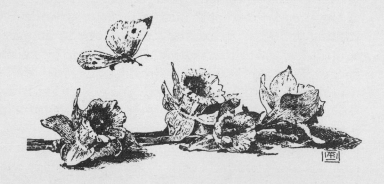

HOW-TO EXPLORATIONS TO TRY

—While feeling ill, emotionally discouraged, or depressed, give yourself the therapy of laughter. Go to a funny movie, watch a funny television show or video tape. At first, you may not feel like laughing— laugh anyway, as deeply as possible— for at least ten minutes. Do this as often as you need it, even several times a day. Take note; is your experience similar to the observations of Norman Cousins?

—You might, like Herbert Howe, set yourself a challenging goal—one that will require effort and growth on your part. This goal need not be physical. Try to do or achieve something you've always felt incapable of—but yet wanted. Spend some time each day on that goal, taking your progress in small, persistent steps.

—Select something about which you've been procrastinating. When you feel like putting it off again, *do it anyway!* What does it feel like, when you have completed this task?

—Listen with complete attention to your favorite music. As you do so, do your best to immerse yourself in the sound. If you feel a chill up your spine, that's an indication of the presence of Endorphins.

—If you find yourself deriving joy from only one thing, person, or situation, you need to diversify your happiness—in order to prepare for life's inevitable change. Broaden your scope of relationships toward the people in your life—and to the world around you.

—Try to be conscious of the times you harbor bitterness, resentment, or anger—especially over events of the past. As these issues arise, find ways to release these biochemical addictions. An honest, open-minded journal can help. Seek counseling from a trusted advisor or cleric of your faith. Focus on the healing that forgiveness can bring you. See if forgiveness is an Endorphin trigger for you.

—If you find that you are an introverted, shy person who prefers books, television, or quiet, reflective kinds of activity, stimulate the opposite response by developing new ways to relate to others and the active world around you. Remember that dendrite growth was not found in a solitary cage.

—If you are an active, extroverted person, who enjoys the stimulus of intereaction with your friends and family, you may notice that you hate to be alone, or feel markedly lonely while by yourself. Develop ways to be at peace and centered in quietude. You will benefit from untapped, parasympathetic Endorphins derived from relaxation, meditation, and contemplative activities. Keep a journal of your thoughts and feelings.

—From the writing of Rev. Flower A. Newhouse, founder of The Christward Ministry and Questhaven Retreat, we can borrow an uplifting discipline to use while walking in nature. Focus each of your five senses, one at a time, as you would tune into five separate stations on a radio. Take time to appreciate each awareness fully. Then, modulate all five senses, trying to tune into all of them simultaneously. This is an excellent Endorphin trigger—one that can help you attain a heightened awareness.

—No matter how we wish to define God, each of us can find meaning in life through an attuned Oneness with Creation. What gives you your highest joy? Euphoric Endorphins—part of the bio-electrical charge we call life—are flowing during your most profound times of awareness—your *mystical* experiences. What impressions give you a sense of deep meaning in your life? The answers to these questions help you define your place in Creation. Seek your own ongoing experience of joy—celebrate—become addicted to *loving life*, as life flows through and around you.

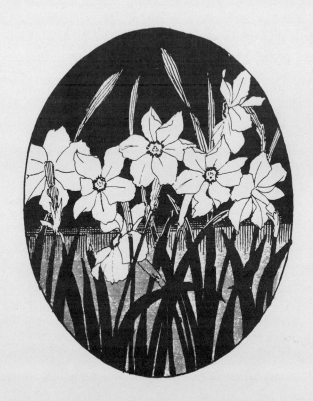

Pleasure Connection

..Build thee more stately mansions, O my soul,
As the swift seasons roll! Leave thy low-vaulted
past! Let each new temple, nobler than the last,
Shut thee from heaven   with a dome more vast, Till
thou at length art free, Leaving thine outgrown
shell by life's unresting sea!
—Oliver Wendell Holmes

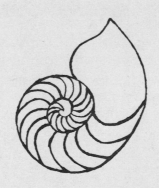

— Epilogue —

A Promise

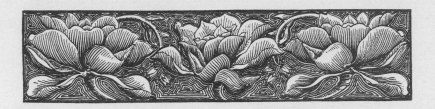

*U*pon discovering a chambered nautilis shell, Oliver Wendell Holmes described his own inspiration—a heightened awareness about the beauty of life. To the poet, the shell became a symbol of an ongoing, ever-upward flow of life. To us, this stanza of Holmes's poem reflects an insight which illumines our own explorations and discoveries.

Reflect upon the eustress of Endorphins—yet another heightened awareness. During eustress, the present moment of experience is filled with a sense of wholeness. There is no feeling of separation at these times. The body and mind, indeed the body and the spirit, are one. This heightened awareness has been described by poets, mystics, and philosophers for millenia.

Pleasure Connection

We may believe that this special experience is for someone else, that we are just ordinary folk, playing out an average, uninspired life-span. But are sages truly a different breed? A potential brain biochemistry exists within everyone. Eustress is an experience we all encounter. Might we each have a potential to leave an outworn shell behind—to discover that the height of joy and wholeness may be the very destination of our Endorphin explorations?

Are bio-electrical Endorphins part of a vast realm of energy that bridges the chasm between our physical bodies and the essence of Spirit?

If the bio-electricity within us is potential for a fine-tuned frequency response, what other currents may be waiting for the receptivity of our own brain's abilities to tune into them? Radio and television waves existed long before amplifiers and tuners were designed.

Radio waves were simply potential transmissions until the radio's receptive capability brought this potential to our reality. Does the Music of the Spheres wait like a radio wave for our own brain's bio-electricity to be tuned, receptive by our appreciation, choice, and focus? Does the earth's vast beauty harbor potential for us to become bio-electrical amplifiers, reverberating with joy? Do Angels sing harmonies just beyond a potential fine-tuning of our bio-electrical hearing?

Might our contemplations conceive of a Great Divinity who created Endorphins in us so that we might, in His Own Image, reverberate to and resonate within the euphoric Beauty of His Creation?

Epilogue

These are thoughts made relevant to Now by the wonderful discoveries of Endorphins and other brain biochemicals, and the promise that ongoing research holds out to our becoming. "Build thee more stately mansions, O my soul!"

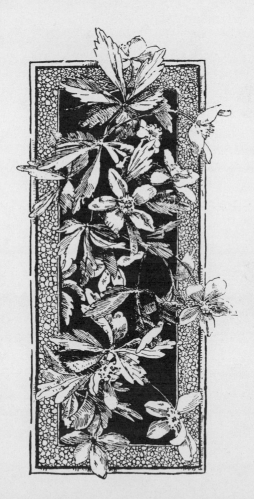

— Glossary —

—ADRENOCORTICOTROPHIC HORMONE, or ACTH—
A hormone secreted from the pituitary gland. ACTH is involved in the body's immune-system maintenance.

—AUTONOMIC NERVOUS SYSTEM—
A part of the nervous system which was thought, until recently, to be concerned with control of involuntary bodily functions, including glands, smooth muscle tissue and the heart. Current research points to potential voluntary control, also.

—AXON—
The branching, limb-like part of a neuron (brain and/or nerve cell) which transmits nerve impulses from the cell's body to other neurons.

—BETA-ENDORPHIN—
A specific Endorphin arising from the pituitary gland. Dr. Choh Hao Li discovered Beta-Endorphin occurring beside ACTH in a longer pituitary peptide chain.

—BURNOUT—
Once considered a slang term, burnout is widely recognized as a condition felt when one is highly stressed, or distressed for prolonged periods of time. Burnout is characterized by a feeling of apathy which has replaced a previous sense of zeal, or caring.

—CORTEX—
The outermost layer of the brain, generally understood as the area responsible for conscious-thought.

—DENDRITES—
The term for the outermost twig-like branches of neurons. Dendrites are receivers of nerve impulses from axons. They are now known to grow in response to stimulus.

—DISEASE—
Literally the lack of ease; a condition which departs from health; illness in general.

—DISTRESS—
A specific kind of stress characterized by mental, emotional, and/or physical strain imposed by pain, worry, and anxiety.

—ENDORPHINS—
The general term coined by Dr. Eric Simon for a family of brain biochemicals that relieve pain and create euphoria.

—ENKEPHALINS—
A scientific term for Endorphins. Also a specific Endorphin discovered and named by Dr. John Hughes.

—ENRICHMENT—
Given an improved definition through the discussions in this book—a quality of life which includes full, appreciative awareness of the diversity which life has to offer.

—EUPHORIA—
A feeling of well-being, happiness, pleasure, now known to be created by naturally occurring biochemicals in the body.

Glossary

—EUSTRESS—
A term coined by Dr. Hans Selye to indicate the kind of stress which is good and causes pleasure. It is the type of stress which stimulates euphoria.

—HOMEOSTASIS—
A state of equilibrium or balance within the body.

—HORMONES—
Biochemicals created in a gland or organ of the body, which then circulate within the bloodstream to other parts of the body. Hormones are messengers—communicating the need for functional activity.

—IMMUNITY—
The condition of the body's ability to maintain health by defending against injury or disease, particularly from bacteria, parasites, and/or poisons.

—LIMBIC BRAIN—
The middle layer of the brain. According to Dr. Paul MacLean's theory, it is the seat of conscious and unconscious emotions.

—LYMPHOCYTE—
A specific kind of white blood cell circulating in the bloodstream as one of the body's first defenses against disease.

—NALOXONE—
A chemical antidote, known to reverse the effects of drugs like morphine. Now it is also used as a test for the action of Endorphins in the body.

—NEURON—
The scientific term for brain and nerve cells.

—PARASYMPATHETIC—
The resting, relaxation phase of the autonomic nervous system.

—PHASE RELATIONSHIP—
A term used by audio engineers to describe the unified sound effect which stereo speakers can achieve when placed and balanced properly.

—PLACEBO—
Previously defined as a sugar pill, saline injection, or "fake" therapy given for an imaginary pain. Endorphin research broadens the definition to include a natural biochemical response activated by *belief* in a given therapy.

—POSTPARTUM DEPRESSION—
A special kind of depression often experienced by mothers after delivery. Research now implicates a shift in the balance of Endorphins, which have been high throughout the recent pregnancy.

—PSYCHONEUROIMMUNOLOGY—
A medical sub-specialty which studies the connections between the mind (psycho), brain (neuro), and the body's ability to defend against disease (immuno).

—RECEPTOR SITES—
A scientific term used to define specialized areas on the cells of our body. Receptor sites are likened to "keyholes" which receive biochemical "keys." Endorphins are our example of biochemical keys which "lock" into receptor sites and, thereby, work in our bodies.

—REPTILIAN BRAIN—
The innermost, deepest layer of our brain, also called the *brainstem*. According to Dr. Paul MacLean's theory, it is the brain responsible for our survival—both physically and psychologically—containing its own set of unconscious instincts.

Glossary

—STIMULUS—

The flow of bio-electricity transmitted to the brain and nervous system by impulses from our five senses.

—STRESS—

Previously defined as a intense strain or pressure, the term *stress* has been recently refined by Dr. Hans Selye, who first studied its effects upon the body (reference "distress" and "eustress"). Stress can be mental, emotional, physical, or a combination of the three. Endorphins are often triggered by stress.

—SYMPATHETIC—

The active, "fight or flight" phase of the autonomic nervous system.

—SYNAPSE—

A bio-electrical impulse or chemical "flash" momentarily created in the space between the dendrites found throughout the brain and nervous system. Nerve impulses travel through the flow of one synapse to another.

❈ ❈ ❈

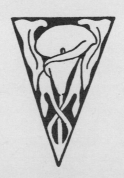

— Bibliography —

We have included, whenever possible, the universities and places in which Endorphin research is being done. This is to give you, the reader, a sense of the width and depth of Endorphin exploration throughout the world.

Introduction

Ardell, Donald B. *High Level Wellness.* Emmaus, Pennsylvania: Rodale Press, 1977.

Davis, Joel. *Endorphins, New Waves in Brain Chemistry.* Garden City, New York: The Dial Press, 1983.

Ellenwood, S. and R.W. Wilson, Michigan State University. "Endorphins and ethics." *Ethics in Science and Medicine,* Vol. 7 (1980), pp. 159-60.

Goldstein, Avram, Addiction Research Foundation, Palo Alto, California. "Opiod peptides: function and significance." *Opiods, Past, Present and Future,* ed. J. Hughes, H.O.J. Collier, M.J. Rarce and M.B. Tyres. London and Philadelphia: Taylor and Francis, 1984, pp. 127-143.

Jaffe, Dennis T. *Healing From Within.* New York: Alfred A. Knopf, 1980.

Maranto, Gina. "The mind within the brain." *Discover,* Vol. 5, No. 5 (May, 1984), pp. 34-43.

Pelletier, Kenneth R. *Holistic Medicine From Stress to Optimum Health.* New York: Delacorte Press, 1979.

Simon, Eric J. New York University Medical Center. "History." *Endorphins, Chemistry, Physiology, Pharmacology and Clinical Relevance,* eds. J.B. Malick, and R.M.S. Bell. New York: Marcel Dekker, Inc., 1982.

Sobel, David S., ed. *Ways of Health, Holistic Approaches*

to *Ancient and Contemporary Medicine.* New York: Harcourt Brace Jovanovich, 1979.

Watson, S. J., et al, Mental Health Research Institute, University of Michigan, Ann Arbor. "Opiod systems: anatomical, physiological and clinical perspectives." *Opiods, Past, Present and Future,* eds. J. Hughes, H.O.J. Collier, M.J. Rarce, and M.B. Tyres. London and Philadelphia: Taylor and Francis, 1984, pp. 145-178.

Weiner, H.M. *Psychobiology and Human Disease.* New York: Elsevier Press, 1977.

Chapter One

Akil, H., D.J. Mayer, and J.C. Liebeskind, Stanford University, Palo Alto, and University of California, Los Angeles. "Antagonism of stimulation produced analgesia by naloxone antagonist." *Science,* Vol. 191 (1976), pp. 961-962.

—————, J. Hughes, and J.D. Barchas, Stanford University, Palo Alto, California. "Enkephalin-like material elevated in ventricular cerebro-spinal fluid of patients after focal stimulation." *Science,* Vol. 201 (1978), pp. 463-465.

Amir, S., Z.W. Brown, and Z. Amit, Concordia University, Quebec, Canada. "The role of Endorphins in stress: evidence and speculations." *Neuroscience and Biobehavioral Reviews,* Vol. 4 (Spring, 1980), pp. 77-81.

Atweh. S.F., and M.J. Kuhar, University of Chicago, Illinois, and Johns Hopkins University, Baltimore, Maryland. "Distribution of physiological significance of opiod receptors in the brain." *British Medical Bulletin,* Vol. 39, No. 1 (1983), pp. 47-52.

Begley, S., J. Carey, and R. Sawhill. "How the brain works." *Newsweek* (February 7, 1983), pp. 40-47.

Benson, Herbert. *The Relaxation Response.* New York: William Morrow and Co., 1975.

Berger, P.A., H. Akil, and J.D. Barchas, Stanford Universi-

Bibliography

ty, Palo Alto, California. "Behavioral pharmacology of the Endorphins." *Annual Reviews of Medicine,* Vol. 33 (1982), pp. 397-415.

Bloom, Floyd E., Salk Institute, La Jolla, California. "Neuropeptides." *Scientific American,* Vol. 254, No. 4 (October 1981), pp. 148-168.

Bolles, R.C. and M.S. Fanselow, University of Washington, Seattle, and Dartmouth College, Hanover, New Hampshire. "Endorphins and behavior." *American Review of Psychology,* Vol. 33 (1982), pp. 87-101.

Bortz, W.M., et al, Stanford University, Palo Alto, California. "Catecholamines, Dopamine and Endorphin levels during extreme exercise." *The New England Journal of Medicine,* Vol. 305 (August 20, 1981), pp. 466-467.

Carr, D., et al, Harvard Medical School, Boston. "Physical conditioning facilitates the exercise-induced secretion of B-Endorphin and B-lipoprotein in women." *New England Journal of Medicine,* Vol. 305 (September 3, 1981), pp. 560-63

————. "Endorphins in contemporary medicine." *Comprehensive Therapy,* Vol. 9, No. 3 (1983), pp. 40-45.

Colt, E.W., D.S.L. Wardlaw, and A.G. Frantz, Columbia University, New York. "The effect of running on plasma B-Endorphin." *Life Science,* Vol. 28 (1981), pp. 1637-1640.

Cox, B.M., et al, Stanford University, Palo Alto, California. "A peptide-like substance that acts like a morphine. 2. Purification and properties." *Life Science,* Vol. 16 (June 15, 1975), pp. 1777-82.

Cuello, A. Claudio, Oxford, England. "Central distribution of opiod peptides." *British Medical Bulletin,* Vol. 39, No. 1 (1983), pp. 11-16.

Davis, B.J., G.D. Burd, and F. Macrides, Worcester Foundation for Experimental Biology, Shrewsbury, Massachusetts. "Localization of Methionine-enkephalin, Substance P and Somatostatin immunoreactivities in the main olfactory bulb of the hamster." *The Journal of*

Comparative Neurology, Vol. 204 (1982), pp. 377-383.

Davis, Joel. *Endorphins, New Waves in Brain Chemistry.* Garden City, New York: The Dial Press, 1983.

Dubois, M., et al, National Institute of Health, Bethesda, Maryland. "Surgical stress in humans is accompanied by an increase in plasma Beta-Endorphin immunoreactivity." *Life Sciences,* Vol. 29 (1981), pp. 1249-1254.

Duggan, A.W., Australian National University, Canberra. "Electrophysiology of opiod peptides and sensory systems." *British Medical Bulletin,* Vol. 39, No.1 (1983), pp. 65-70.

Friedman, Milton. *Type A Behavior and Your Heart.* New York: Alfred A. Knopf, 1974.

Goldstein, A., et al, Stanford University, Palo Alto, California. "Dynorphin-[1-13], an extraordinarily potent opiod peptide." *Proceedings, National Academy of Sciences (U.S.A.),* Vol. 76 (December, 1979), pp. 6666-70.

Greist, J.H., et al, University of Wisconsin, Madison. "Running as treatment for depression." *Comprehensive Psychiatry,* Vol. 20, No. 1 (January/February, 1979), pp. 41-54.

Grossman, A., and L.H. Rees, St. Bartholomew's Hospital, London, England. "The neuroendocrinology of opiod peptides." *British Medical Bulletin,* Vol 39, No. 1 (1983), pp. 83-88.

Guillemin, Roger, Salk Institute, La Jolla, California. "Peptides in the brain: the new endocrinology of a neuron." *Science,* Vol. 202 (October 27, 1978), pp. 390-402.

—————, et al. "The Endorphins: novel peptides of brain and hypophysial origin, with opiate-like activity: biochemical and biologic properties." *Annals of The New York Academy of Sciences,* Vol. 27 (1977), pp. 131-157.

—————, et al. "Characterization of the Endorphins, novel hypothalamic and neurohypophysial peptides with opiate-like activity: evidence that they induce profound behavioral changes."*Psychoneuroendocrino-*

Bibliography

logy, Vol. 2 (1977), pp. 59-62.

Henderson, Graeme, Cambridge, England."Electrophysilogical analysis of opiod action in the central nervous system." *British Medical Bulletin,* Vol. 39, No. 1 (1983), pp. 59-64.

Hughes, J., et al, University of Aberdeen, Scotland. "Identification of two related pentapeptides from the brain with potent opiate agonist activity." *Nature,* Vol. 258 (December 18, 1975), pp. 577-579.

————, and H.W. Kosterlitz, Imperial College of Science and Technology, London, England. "Introduction opiod peptides." *British Medical Bulletin,* Vol 39, No. 1 (1983), pp. 1-3.

Imura, H., et al, Kyoto University, Japan. "Effect of CNS peptides on hypothalamic regulation of pituitary secretion." *Neurosecretion and Brain Peptides,* eds. J.B. Martin, S. Reichlin, and K.L. Bick. New York: Raven Press, 1981.

Iverson, Leslie L., Cambridge, England. "The chemistry of the brain." *Scientific American,* Vol. 241 (September, 1979), pp. 134-139.

Kangawa. K., et al, Miyazaki Medical College, Yiyotake, Japan. "A neo-endorphin: a "big" Leu-enkephalin with potent opiate activity from porcine hypothalamus." *Biochemical and Biophysical Research Communications,* Vol. 86 (January 15, 1979), pp. 153-60.

Kilpatrick, D.L., et al, Roche Institute of Molecular Biology, Nutley, New Jersey. "Rimorphin, a unique, naturally occurring (Leu)enkephalin-containing peptide found in association with Dynorphin and A-neo-endorphin." *National Academy of Sciences (U.S.A.),* Vol. 79 (November, 1982), pp. 6480-83.

King, C., et al, Louisiana State University, New Orleans. "Effects of B-Endorphin and morphine on the sleep-wakefulness behavior of cats." *Sleep,* Vol. 4, No. 3 (1981), pp. 259-262.

Koob, G.F., and F.E. Bloom, Salk Institute, La Jolla, California. "Behavioural effects of opiod peptides." *British Medical Bulletin*, Vol. 39, No.1 (1983), 89-94.

LeRoith, D., et al, National Institute of Mental Health, Bethesda, Maryland. "Corticotropin and B-Endorphin-like materials are native to unicellular organisms." *Proceedings. National Academy of Sciences (U.S.A.)*, Vol. 79 (March, 1982), pp. 2086-90.

McQueen, D.S., University of Edinburg Medical School, Scotland. "Opiod Peptide Interactions with Respiratory and Circulating Systems." *British Medical Bulletin*, Vol. 39, No. 1 (1983), pp. 77-82.

Malick, J.B., and M.S. Bell, eds. *Endorphins: Chemistry, Physiology, Pharmacology and Clinical Relevance.* New York: Marcel Dekker, Inc., 1982.

Mancillas, J.R., et al, Salk Institute, La Jolla, California. "Immunocytochemical localization of Enkephalin and Substance P in retina and eyestalk neurons of lobster." *Nature*, Vol. 239 (October 15, 1981), pp. 376-377.

Markoff, R.A., P. Ryan, and T. Young, University of Hawaii, Honolulu. "Endorphins and mood changes in long-distance running." *Medicine and Science in Sports and Exercise*, Vol. 14, No. 1 (1982), pp. 11-15.

Martin, J.B. *Functions of Neurosecretion and Brain Peptides.* New York: Raven Press, 1981.

Millan, M.J., Max-Planck Institute of Psychiatry, Munich, West Germany. "Stress and endrogenous opiod peptides: a review." *Modern Problems in Pharmacopsychiatry*, eds. T.A. Ban, et al. Basel, Switzerland: S. Kargen, 1981, pp. 49-67.

Miller, R.J., and V.M. Pickel, University of Chicago, Illinois and Cornell Medical College, New York. "The distribution and functions of the Enkephalins." *The Journal of Histochemistry and Cytochemistry*, Vol. 28, No. 8 (1980), pp. 903-917.

Minimino, N., et al, Miyazaki Medical College, Kiyotaka, Japan. "B-neo-endorphin, a new hypothalamic "big" Leuenkephalin of porcine origin: its purification and

Bibliography

the complete amino acid sequence." *Biochemical and Biophysical Research Communications*, Vol. 99 (April 15, 1981), pp. 864-70.

Morgan, W.P. and D.H. Horstman, University of Wisconsin, Madison. "Anxiety reduction following acute physical activity." *Medicine and Science in Sports and Exercise*, Vol. 8 (1976), p. 62.

Ornstein, Robert E. *The Psychology of Consciousness.* San Francisco: W.H. Freeman & Co., 1972.

"Opiate peptides, analgesia and the neuroendocrine system." *British Medical Journal*, No. 6216 (March 15, 1980), pp. 741-742.

Pelletier, Kenneth R. *Mind as Healer, Mind as Slayer, A Holistic Approach To Preventing Stress Disorders.* New York: Dell Publishing Co., 1977.

Pert, Agu, National Institute of Mental Health, Bethesda, Maryland. "The body's own tranquilizers." *Psychology Today*, Vol. 15 (March 9, 1973), pp. 1011-14.

Pickar, D., et al, National Institutes of Health, Bethesda, Maryland. "Response of plasma cortisol and B-Endorphin immunoreactivity to surgical stress." *Psychopharmacology Bulletin*, Vol. 18 (July, 1982), pp. 208-211.

Polak, J.M., and S.R. Bloom, Royal Postgraduate Medical School, London, England. "The diffuse neuroendocrine system." *The Journal of Histochemistry and Cytochemistry*, Vol. 27, No. 10 (1979), pp. 1398-1400.

Pribram, Karl. *Languages of The Brain, Experimental Paradoxes and Principles in Neuropsychology.* Monterey, California: Brooks/Cole Publishing Co., 1977.

Quinby, Brie P. "The fitness fix: why exercise is a great high." *Mademoiselle*, Vol. 88 (March, 1982), p. 94.

Restak, Richard M. *The Brain, The Final Frontier.* New York: Doubleday, 1979.

Schwartz, J.C., and B.P. Roques, U.E.R. des Sciences Pharmaceutiques et Biolgiques, Paris, France. "Opiod peptides as intercellular messengers." *Biomedicine*, Vol. 32 (1980), pp. 169-175.

Selye, Hans. *Stress Without Distress.* New York: Dutton, 1974.

Snyder, Solomon H., Johns Hopkins University, Baltimore, Maryland. "Drug and neurotransmitter receptors in the brain." *Science,* Vol. 224 (April 6, 1984), pp. 22-31.

Stevens, Charles F. "The neuron." *The Brain, A Scientific American Book.* San Francisco: W.H. Freeman & Co., 1979.

Terenius, L., and A. Wahlstrom, University of Uppsala, Sweden. "Morphine-like ligand for opiate receptors in human CSF." *Life Sciences,* Vol. 16 (June 15, 1975), pp. 1759-64.

———. "Antagonism of stimulation produced analgesia by naloxone, a narcotic antagonist." *Science,* Vol. 191 (1976), pp. 961-962.

Tower, Donald B., National Institutes of Health, Bethesda, Maryland. "Epilogue." *Neurosecretions and Brain Peptides,* eds. J.B. Martin, S. Reichlin, and K.L. Bick. New York: Raven Press, 1981, pp. 691-693.

van Praag, H.M., and W.M.A. Verhoeven, University of Utrecht, The Netherlands. "Neuropeptides, a new dimension in biological psychiatry." *Progress in Brain Research, Vol. 53* (1980), pp. 329-47.

Walsh, Roger. *Towards an Ecology of Brain.* New York: Spectrum Publications, Inc., 1981.

Wei, E., University of California, Berkeley. "Enkephalin analogs and physical dependence." *Journal of Pharmacology and Experimental Therapeutics,* Vol. 216 (June, 1981), pp. 12-18.

———, and H. Loh. "Physical dependence on opiate-like peptides." *Science,* Vol. 193 (September 24, 1976), pp. 1262-1263.

Wenyon, Michael. *Understanding Holography.* New York: Arco Publishing Company, Inc., 1978.

Williams, J.T. and W. Zieglansberger, Max-Planck Institute of Psychiatry, Munich, West Germany. "Neurons in the frontal cortex of the rat carry multiple opiate re-

Bibliography

ceptors." *Brain Research,* Vol. 226 (1981), pp. 304-308.

Wise, S.P. and M. Herkenham, National Institute of Mental Health, Bethesda, Maryland. "Opiate receptor distribution in the cerebral cortex of the rhesus monkey." *Science,* Vol. 218 (October, 22, 1982), pp. 387-92.

Zetler, G., Medical School of Lubeck, Federal Republic of Germany. "Active peptides in the nervous tissue: historical perspectives." *Advances in Biochemical Psychopharmacology* , *Vol. 18,* eds. E. Costa, and M. Trabucchi. New York: Raven Press, 1978, pp. 1-13.

The Diagram Group. *The Brain, A User's Manual.* New York: Perigee Books, 1982.

Chapter Two

Antelman, S.M., and N. Rowland, University of Pittsburg, Pennsylvania. "Endrogenous opiates and stress-induced eating."*Science,* Vol. 214 (December, 1981), pp. 1149-50.

Ball, Aimee Lee. "To: Candace Pert for: brain power." *Redbook Magazine,* Vol.153, No. 5 (September, 1979), p. 56.

Beecher, Henry K., American Mediterranean Theater of Operations, WWII. "Pain in men wounded in battle." *Annals of Surgery,* Vol. 123, No. 1 (1946), pp. 96-105.

Berger, P.A., and J.D. Barchas, Stanford University, Palo Alto, California. "Studies of B-Endorphin in psychiatric patients." *Annals New York Academy of Sciences,* Vol. 398 (December 20, 1982), pp. 448-459.

Bloom, F.E., et al, University of California, San Diego, and the Salk Institute, La Jolla, California. "B-Endorphin: cellular localization, electrophysiological and behavioral effects." *Advances in Biochemical Psychopharmacology, Vol. 18,* eds. E. Costa, and M. Trabucchi. New York: Raven Press, 1978.

————. "Endorphins as mediators of ethanol actions: multidisciplinary tests." *Advances in Endrogenous and Exogenous Opiods; Proceedings* (July, 26-30, 1981), p. 226 ff.

Blum, K., M.G. Hamilton, and J.E. Wallace, University of Texas, San Antonio, and University of Western Ontario, London, Ontario, Canada. "Alcohol and opiates: a review of common neurochemical and behavioral mechanisms." *Alcohol and Opiates, Neurochemical and Behavioral Mechanisms,* ed. by K. Blum. New York: Academic Press, Inc., 1977.

Brown, D.R. and S.G. Holtzman, Emory University, Atlanta, Georgia. "Suppression of deprivation induced food and water intake in rats and mice by nalaxone." *Pharmacology, Biochemistry and Behavior,* Vol. 11 (1979), pp. 567-73.

Davis, K.L., et al, Palo Alto V.A. Medical Center, California, and Bronx V.A. Medical Center, New York. "Neuroendocrine and neurochemical measurements in depression." *American Journal of Psychiatry,* Vol. 138, No. 12 (December, 1981), pp. 1555-1561.

Dubos, Rene. *The Mirage of Health.* New York: Doubleday/Anchor Books, 1959.

Eihnhorn, D., J.B. Young, and L. Landsberg, Harvard Medical School, Boston, Massachusetts. "Hypotensive effect of fasting: possible involvement of the sympathetic nervous system and endrogenous opiates." *Science,* Vol. 217 (August 20, 1982), pp. 727-729.

Facchinetti, F., et al, Universities of Siena, Messina, Perugia, and Cagliari, Italy. "Opiod plasma levels during labor." *Gynecologic and Obstetric Investigation,* Vol. 13 (1982), pp. 1555-163.

Forman, L.J., et al, Michigan State University, East Lansing. "Immunoreactive B-Endorphin in the plasma, pituitary and hypothalamus of young and old male rats." *Neurobiology of Aging,* Vol. 2 (1982), pp. 281-284.

Furuhashi, N., et al, Tohoku University School of Medicine, Sendai, Japan. "Plasma Adrenocorticotrophic Hormone, Beta-Lipotropin, and Beta-Endorphin in the human fetus at delivery." *Gynecologic and Obstetric Investigation,* Vol. 14 (1982), pp. 236-239.

Bibliography

Gilman, A.G., et al, University of California, San Diego. "B-Endorphin enhances lymphocyte proliferative responses." *Proceedings of the National Academy of Sciences, (U.S.A.)*, Vol. 79 (July, 1982), pp. 4226-4230.

Goodlin, R.C., University of Nebraska, Omaha. "Nalaxone and its possible relationship to fetal Endorphin levels and fetal distress." *American Journal of Obstetrics and Gynecology*, Vol. 139 (1981), pp. 16-19.

Halbreich, U., and J. Endicott, Montefiore Medical Center, Bronx, New York. "Possible involvement of Endorphin withdrawal or imbalance in specific premenstrual syndromes and postpartum depression." *Medical Hypotheses*, Vol. 7 (1981), pp. 1045-1058.

Hutchinson, J.S., et al, University of Melbourne, Australia. "Effects of bromocriptine on blood pressure and plasma B-Endorphin in spontaneously hypertensive rats." *Clinical Science*, Vol. 61 (1981), pp. 343s-345s.

Johnson, H.M., et al, University of Texas, Galveston. "Regulation of the in vitro antibody response by neuroendocrine hormones." *Proceedings of the National Academy of Sciences (U.S.A.)*, Vol. 79, (July, 1982), pp. 4171-4174.

Judd, L.L., et al, University of California, San Diego. "Endrogenous opiod mechanism in neuroendocrine regulation in normal and psychopathological states." *Psychopharmacology Bulletin*, Vol. 18, No. 3 (July 1982), pp. 204-207.

Konturek, Stanislaw J., Institute of Physiology, Krakow, Poland. "Opiates and the gastrointestinal tract." *American Journal of Gastroenterology*, Vol. 74 (1980), pp. 285-291.

Kovacs. G.L., G. Telegdy, and D. De Weid, University Medical School, Szeged, Hungary, and University of Utrecht, The Netherlands. "Selective attenuation of passive avoidance behavior by microinjection of B-LPH 62-77 and B-LPH 66-77 into the nucleus accumbens in rats." *Neuropharmacology*, Vol. 21 (1982), pp. 451-455.

Kuich, T.E., and D. Zimmerman, Mayo Graduate School of Medicine, Rochester, Minnesota. "Endorphins, ventilatory control and sudden infant death syndrome—a review and synthesis." *Medical Hypotheses*, Vol. 7 (1981), pp. 1231-1240.

Lipsitz, L.A., et al, Hebrew Rehabilitation Center for the Aged, Boston, Massachusetts. "Postprandial reduction in blood pressure in elderly." *New England Journal of Medicine*, Vol. 39, No. 2 (July 14, 1983), pp. 81-83.

McCain, H.W., et al, Fairleigh Dickinson University School of Dentistry, Hackensack, New Jersey. "B-Endorphin modulates human immune activity via nonopiate receptor mechanisms." *Life Sciences*, Vol. 31 (1982), pp. 1619-1624.

Mandenoff, A., et al, Laboratoire de Nutrition Humaine, Paris, France, and Temple University, Philadelphia, Pennsylvania. "Endrogenous opiates and energy balance." *Science*, Vol. 215 (March, 1982), pp. 1536-37.

Margules, David L., Temple University, Philadelphia, Pennsylvania. "Obesity and the hibernation response." *Psychology Today*, Vol. 13, No. 10 (October 1979), p. 136.

Miranda, H., G. Bustos, and H. Lara, Pontifica Universidad Catolica, Santiago, Chile. "Chronic ethanol administration induces tolerance to morphine and to B-Endorphin responses in the rat vas deferens." *European Journal of Pharmacolgy*, Vol. 87 (1983), pp. 291-296.

Morley, J.E., and A.S. Levine, University of Minnesota, Minneapolis. "The role of the endrogenous opiate as regulators of appetite." *The American Journal of Clinical Nutrition*, Vol. 35 (April 1982), pp. 757-761.

————. "Stress-induced eating is mediated through endrogenous opiates."*Science*, Vol. 209 (September, 1980), pp. 1259-1260.

————. "The neuroendocrine control of appetite: the role of the endrogenous opiates, Cholecystokinin, TRH, GABA, and the diazepam receptor." *Life Sciences*, Vol. 27,

Bibliography

No. 5 (1980), pp. 355-368.

————. "The endocrinology of the opiates and opiod peptides." *Metabolism*, Vol. 30, No. 2 (February, 1981), pp. 195-204.

Moss, I.R., and E.M. Scarpelli, Albert Einstein College of Medicine, Bronx, New York. "B-Endorphin central depression of respiration and circulation." *Journal of Applied Physiology*, Vol. 50 (1981), pp. 1011-1016.

"Nicotine spurs Endorphins." *Brain/Mind Bulletin*, Vol 9, No. 4 (January 23, 1984), p. 3.

North, R.A., and T.M. Egan, Massachusetts Institute of Technology, Cambridge. "Actions and distributions of opiod peptides in peripheral tissues." *British Medical Bulletin*, Vol. 39, No. 1 (1983), pp. 71-75.

Pert, Agu, National Institute of Mental Health, Bethesda, Maryland. "The body's own tranquilizers." *Psychology Today*, Vol. 15, No. 9 (September, 1981), p. 100.

Petty, M.A., J.M.A. Sitsen, and W. DeJong, University of Utrecht, The Netherlands. "B-Endorphin, and endrogenous depressor agent in the rat?" *Clinical Science*, Vol. 61 (1981), pp. 339s-342s.

Recant, L., et al, National Institute of Mental Health, Bethesda, Maryland, "Naltrexone reduces weight gain, alters B-Endorphin and reduces insulin output from pancreatic islets of genetically obese mice." *Peptides*, Vol. 1, No. 4 (1980), pp. 309-314.

Reus, Victor, Langley Porter Institute, San Francisco, California. "Neuropeptide modulation of opiate and ETOH tolerance and dependence." *Medical Hypotheses*, Vol. 6, No. 11 (1980), pp. 1141-1148.

Riley, A.L., D.A. Zellner, and H.J. Duncan, The American University, Washington, D.C. "The role of Endorphins in animal learning and behavior." *Neuroscience and Biobehavioral Reviews*, Vol. 4 (September, 20, 1979), pp. 69-76.

Risch, S.C., et al, University of California, San Diego. "Elevated plasma B-Endorphin concentrations in de-

pression   and cholinergically sensitive release mechanisms *Psychopharmacology   Bulletin*, Vol. 18, No. 3
(July, 1982), pp. 211-215.

—————, et al, National Institute of Mental Health, Be-
thesda, Maryland, and University of California, San
Diego.   "Mood and behavioral effects of physiotigmine
on humans are accompanied by elevations in plasma B-
Endorphin and cortisol."   *Science*, Vol. 209, No. 26
(September, 1980), pp. 1545-46.

Schwartz, T.B. "Naloxone and weight reduction: an exercise in introspection." *Transactions of Amercian Clinical and Clinitological Association*, Vol. 92 (1981), pp.
103-110.

Selye, Hans. *The Stress of Life.* New York: Mc Graw-Hill
Book Co., 1956.

Shealy, C. Norman. "Preventive, stress, and energy medicine." Workshop presented at *Awards for Excellence in
Health and Education.*   Association for Holistic
Health Conference. Irvine, California. September,
1985.

Sicuteri, F. "Opiods, pregnancy and the disappearance of
headache." *Headache*, Vol. 20 (July, 1980), pp. 220-1.

Simon, Eric J., New York University, New York. "Opiate
receptors and Endorphins: possible relevance to narcotic
addiction." *Advances in Substance and Alcohol Abuse*,
Vol.1 (Fall, 1981), pp. 13-32.

Smith, G.P., and J. Gibbs, Cornell Medical School, New
York. "Brain-gut peptides and the control of food in-
take." *Neurosecretion and Brain Peptides*, eds. J.B.
Martin, S. Reichlin, and K.L. Bick. New York: Raven
Press, 1981.

Steinbrook, R.A., et al, Harvard Medical School, Boston,
Massachusetts. "Dissociation of plasma and cerebrospi-
nal fluid Beta-Endorphin-like immunoactivity levels
during pregnancy and parturition." *Anesthesia and
Analgesia*, Vol. 61, No. 11 (November, 1982), pp. 893-
897.

Bibliography

Terenius, Lars, University of Uppsala, Sweden. "Endorphins—the first three years." *American Heart Journal* , Vol. 98, No. 6 (December, 1979), pp. 681-683.

Thornhill, J.A., K.E. Cooper, and W.L. Veale, University of Calgary, Alberta. "Core temperature changes following administration of naloxone and naltrexone to rats exposed to hot and cold ambient temperatures. Evidence for the physiological role of Endorphins in hot and cold acclimatization." *Journal of Pharmacy and Pharmacology*, Vol. 32 (December, 12, 1979), pp. 427-430.

Tregear, G.W., and J.P. Coghian, University of Melbourne, Victoria, Australia. "Alcohol addiction: are the endrogenous opiods involved?" *Australia/New Zealand Journal of Medicine*, Vol. 11 (1981), pp. 118-122.

Wei, E., University of California, Berkeley. "Enkephalin analogs and physical dependence." *Journal of Pharmacology and Experimental Therapeutics*, Vol. 216 (June, 1981), pp. 12-18.

_____, and H. Loh. "Physical dependence on opiate-like peptides." *Science*, Vol. 193 (September, 24, 1976), pp. 1262-63.

Chapter Three

Agnoli, A, et al, University of L'Aquila, and University of Rome, Italy. "On the etiopathogenenesis of migraine: a possible link between the amines and Endorphin hypotheses." *Advances in Neurology*, eds. M. Critchley, et al. New York: Raven Press, 1982.

Akil, H., et al, University of Michigan, Ann Arbor. "Characterization of multiple forms of Beta-Endorphin in pituitary and brain: effect of stress." *Advances in Biochemical Psychopharmacology*, Vol. 3 (1982), pp. 61-67.

Ambinder, R.F., and M.M. Schuster, Johns Hopkins School of Medicine, Baltimore, Maryland. "Endorphins: new gut peptides with a familiar face." *Gastroenterology*,

Vol. 77 (November, 1979), pp. 1132-1140.

Banthrop, R.W., et al, University of New South Wales, Sydney, Australia. "Depressed lymphocyte function after bereavement."*Lancet*, Vol. 1, No. 8016 (April 16, 1977), pp. 834-36.

Beecher, Henry K., Harvard Medical School, Boston, Massachusetts. "The powerful placebo." *Journal of the American Medical Association*, Vol. 159 (1955), pp. 1602-1606.

"Beta-Endorphin as arthritis culprit." *Science News*, Vol. 119 (June 6, 1981), pp. 358-359.

"Brain switch for stress." *Science News*, Vol. 9, No. 6 (June, 1982), p.91.

Della Bella, D., et al, Zambom S. P. A. Research Laboratories, Bresso-Milan, and University of Florence, Italy. " Endorphins in the pathogenesis of headache." *Advances in Neurology*, eds. M. Critchley, et al. New York: Raven Press, 1982.

Ferri, S., et al, Universities of Bologna and Milan, Italy. "Interplay between opiod peptides and pituitary hormones." *Regulatory Peptides: From Molecular Biology to Function*, eds. E. Costa, and M. Trabucchi. New York: Raven Press, 1982.

Fields, Howard L., University of California, San Francisco. "An Endorphin-mediated analgesia system: experimental and clinical observations." *Neurosecretion and Brain Peptides*, eds. J.B. Martin, S. Reichlin, and K.L. Bick. New York: Raven Press, 1981.

Fiore, Neil. "Stress management." Lecture at *The Healing Brain.* University of California, San Francisco, 1980.

Gambert, S.R., et al, Medical College of Wisconsin, Milwaukee. "Thyroid hormone regulation of central nervous system, Beta-Endorphin and ACTH."*Hormone and Metabolic Research*, Vol. 12 (1980), pp. 345-346.

Glasser, Ronald J. *The Body is A Hero.* New York: Random House, 1976.

Guillemin, R., et al, Salk Institute, La Jolla, California.

Bibliography

"B-Endorphin and Adrenocorticotrophin are secreted concomitantly by the pituitary gland." *Science*, Vol. 197 (September 10, 1977), pp. 1367-69.

Herz, A., and M.J. Millan, Max-Planck Institute for Psychiatry, Munich, West Germany. "Opiod peptides in the hypothalamic-pituitary axis., Opiod peptides: function and significance."*Opiods, Past, Present and Future*, eds. J. Hughes, H.O.J. Collier, M.J. Rarce, and M.B. Tyres. London and Philadephia: Taylor and Francis, 1984.

Izquierdo, Ivan, Departamento de Bioquimica, RS, Brazil, "Effect of naloxone and morphine on various forms of memory in the rat: possible role of endogenous opiate mechanisms in memory consolidation." *Psychopharmacology*, Vol. 66 (July, 1979), 199-203.

Jacob, J., Pasteur Institute, Paris, France. "Endrogenous morphines and pain control." *Panminerva Medica*, Vol. 24 (1982), pp. 155-159.

Katz, R.J., K.A. Roth, and K. Schmaltz, Mental Health Research Institute, University of Michigan, Ann Arbor. "Endrogenous opiates as mediators of activation and coping." *Endrogenous and Exogenous Opiate Agonists and Antogonists*, ed. E.L. Way. Oxford, England: Pergamon Press, 1980.

Kay, N., J. Allen, and J.E. Morley, University of Minnesota, Minneapolis. "Endorphins stimulate normal human peripheral blood lymphocyte natural killer activity." *Life Sciences*, Vol. 35, No. 1 (1984), pp. 53-59.

Kreiger, D.T., H. Yamaguchi, H., and A.S. Liotta, Mt. Sinai School of Medicine, New York. "Human plasma, ACTH, Lipoprotein, and Endorphin." *Neurosecretion and Brain Peptides*. New York: Raven Press, 1981, pp. 541-556.

Levine, J., N.C. Gordon, and H.F. Fields, University of California, San Francisco. "The mechanism of placebo analgesia." *Lancet*, Vol. 2, No. 8091 (September 23, 1978), pp. 654-657.

Li, C.H., and D. Chung, University of California, San Francisco. "Isolation and structure of an untriakontapeptide with opiate activity from camel pituitary glands." *Proceedings, National Academy of Sciences (U.S.A.),* Vol. 73 (April 1976), pp. 1145-48.

Loh, Y.P., and L.L. Loriaus, National Institutes of Health, Bethesda, Maryland. "Adrocorticotrophic Hormone, B-lipotropin and Endorphin-related peptides in health and disease." *Journal of the American Medical Association,* Vol. 247, No. 7 (February 19, 1982), pp. 1033-34.

Luttinger, D., C.B. Nemeroff, and A.J. Prange, University of North Carolina, Chapel Hill. "The effects of neuropeptides on discrete-trial conditioned avoidance responding."*Brain Research,* Vol. 237 (1982), pp. 183-92.

McGaugh, J.L., et al, University of California, Irvine, and The Hague, The Netherlands. "Role of neurohormones as modulators of memory storage." *Regulatory Peptides: From Molecular Biology to Function,* eds. E. Costa, and M. Trabucchi. New York: Raven Press, 1982.

MacClean, Paul, National Institute of Mental Health, Bethesda, Maryland. "Cerebral Evolution and Emotional Processes: New Findings on the Striatal Complex." *Annals of the New York Academy of Sciences,* Vol. 193 (August 25, 1972), pp.137-49.

—————. "On the Evolution of Three Mentalities." *New Dimensions in Psychiatry: A World View, Vol. II,* eds. S. Arieti, and G. Chzanowki. New York: John Wiley & Sons, 1977.

Maier, S.F., and M. Laudenslager, University of Colorado, Boulder, and University of Denver, Colorado. "Stress and health: exploring the links." *Psychology Today,* Vol. 19, No. 8 (August, 1985), pp. 44-49.

Pelletier, Kenneth R. "Corporate health promotion programs." Workshop presented at *Awards for Excellence in Health and Education.* Association For Holistic Health Conference, Irvine, California. September, 1985.

Bibliography

Perry, S., and G. Heidrich, Cornell University Medical Center, New York. "Placebo response: myth and matter." *American Journal of Nursing*, Vol. 81, No. 4 (April, 1981), pp. 720-725.

Pert, Agu, National Institute of Mental Health, Bethesda Maryland. "Mechanisms of opiate analgesia and the role of Endorphins in pain suppression." *Advances in Neurology*, eds. M. Critchley, et al. New York: Raven Press, 1982.

Pickar, D., et al, National Institutes of Health, Bethesda, Maryland. "Response of plasma cortisol and B-Endorphin immunoreactivity to surgical stress." *Psychopharmacology Bulletin*, Vol. 18 (July, 1982), pp. 208-211.

Rheingold, Howard. "Endorphins: an emotional story." *Esquire*, Vol. 99, No. 5 (May, 1983), pp. 140-142.

Rigter, H., et al, University of California, Irvine. "Enkephalin and fear-motivated behavior." *Proceedings, National Academy of Sciences (U.S.A.)*, Vol. 77, No. 6 (June, 1980), pp. 3729-3723.

Selye, Hans. *Stress Without Distress*. New York: Dutton, 1974.

—————. *The Stress of Life.* New York: Mc Graw-Hill Book Co., 1956.

Simonton, O.C., S. Matthews-Simonton, and J. Creighton. *Getting Well Again*, Los Angeles: J.P. Tarcher, Inc., 1978.

Solomon, G.F., A.A. Amkraut, and P. Kasper, Stanford University, Palo Alto, California. "Immunity, emotions, and stress." *Annals of Clinical Research*, Vol. 6 (1974), pp. 313-322.

—————, and R.H. Moos, Stanford University, Palo Alto, California. "Emotions, immunity and disease." *Archives of General Psychiatry*, Vol. 11 (1964), pp. 657-674.

Stein, L. and J.D. Belluzzi, University of California, Irvine. "Brain Endorphins: possible role in reward and memory

Pleasure   Connection

formation." *Federation Proceedings*, Vol. 38, No. 11 (October, 1979), pp. 2468-2472.

Stewart, Donald. "Turning on the Endorphins." *American Pharmacology*, Vol. NS20, No. 10 (October, 1980), pp. 50-54.

Summerfield, John A., National Institutes of Health, Bethesda, Maryland. "Pain, itch, and Endorphins." *British Journal of Dermatology*, Vol. 105 (1981), pp. 725-726.

Terenius, Lars, University of Uppsala, Sweden. "Significance of Endorphins in endrogenous antinociception." *Advances in Biochemical Psychopharmacology*, Vol. 18, eds. E. Costa, and M. Trabucchi. New York: Raven Press, 1978.

_____. "Endorphins—the first three years." *American Heart Journal*, Vol. 98, No. 6 (December, 1979), pp. 681-683.

Teschemacher, H., et al, Pharmakologischis Institut der Justus Liebig-Universitat Giessen, Lahn-Geissen, West Germany. "Plasma levels of B-Endorphin/B-lipoprotein in humans under stress." *Endrogenous and exogenous opiate agonists and antagonists*, ed. E.L. Way. Oxford, England: Pergamon Press, 1980.

"What you see is what you eat."*Family Weekly*, (February 8, 1981), p. 30.

Chapter Four

Belluzzi, J.D. and L. Stein, University of California, Irvine. "Brain Endorphins: possible role in long-term memory." *Annals New York Academy of Sciences*, Vol. 398 (1982), pp. 221-229.

Clement-Jones, V., and G.M. Besser, St. Bartholomew's Hospital, London, England. "Clinical perspectives in opiod peptides." *British Medical Bulletin*, Vol. 39, No. 1 (1983), pp. 95-100.

Connor, J. R., and M.C. Diamond, University of California,

220

Bibliography

Berkeley. "A comparison of dendritic spine number and type on pyramidal neuron of the visual cortex of old adult rats from social and isolated environments." *Journal of Comparative Neurology*, Vol. 210 (1982), pp. 99-106.

Diamond, M.C. and J.R. Connor, University of California, Berkeley. "A search for the potential of the aging cortex." *Brain Neurotransmitters and Receptors in Aging and Age Related Disorders.* New York: Raven Press, 1981.

Dupont, A, et al, Le Centre Hospitalier de l'Universite Laval, Quebec, Canada, and Centre De Recherches, Romainville, France. "Age-related changes in central nervous system Enkephalins and Substance P." *Life Sciences*, Vol. 29 (1981), pp. 2317-2322.

"Endorphins through the eye of a needle?" *Lancet*, Vol. 8218 (February 28, 1981), pp. 480-481.

Gambert, S.R., et al, Medical College of Wisconsin, Milwaukee. "Age-related changes in central nervous system Beta-Endorphin and ACTH." *Neuroendocrinology*, Vol. 31 (1980), pp. 252-255.

Han, J., et al, Beijing Medical College, Beijing China, and University of Uppsala, Sweden. "Enkephalin and B-Endorphin as mediators of electro-acupuncture analgesia in rabbits: an antiserum microinjection study." *Regulatory Peptides: From Molecular Biology to Function*, eds. E. Costa and M. Trabucchi. New York: Raven Press, 1982.

Hughes, J., et. al, Imperial College, London, England. "Opiod peptides: aspects of their origin, release and metabolism." *Journal of Experimental Biology*, Vol. 89 (1980), pp. 239-255.

Hopson, Janet L."A love affair with the brain: conversation with Marian Diamond." *Psychology Today*, Vol. 18, No. 11 (November, 1984), pp. 62-73.

Hosobuchi, Y., T.F. Adams, and R. Linchitz, University of California, San Francisco. "Pain relief by electrical stimulation of the central grey matter in humans and its reversal by naloxone." *Science*, Vol. 197 (1976), p. 961.

Kastin, A.J., et al, Tulane University, New Orleans, Louisiana and East Tennessee State University, Johnson City. "Neonatal administration of Met-enkephalin facilitates maze performance in adult rats." *Pharmacology, Biochemistry and Behavior*, Vol. 13 (October,1980), pp. 883-886.

Katz, R.J., University of Michigan Medical Center, Ann Arbor. "Exploration as a functional correlate of Endorphins." *Journal of Theoretical Biology*, Vol. 77 (1979), pp. 537-538.

Kavaliers, M., M. Hirst, and G.C. Teskey, University of Western Ontario, London, Ontario, Canada. "Aging, opiod analgesia and the pineal gland."*Life Sciences*, Vol. 32, No. 19 (1983), pp. 2279-2287.

Maranto, Gina. "The mind within the brain." *Discover*, Vol. 5, No. 5 (May, 1984), pp. 34-43.

Montagu, Ashley. *Touching: the Human Significance of Skin.* New York: Columbia University Press, 1971.

Oyle, Irving. *The Healing Mind.* Millbrae, California: Celestial Arts, 1975.

Riley, A.L., D.A. Zellner, and H.J. Duncan, The American University, Washington D.C. "The role of Endorphins in animal learning and behavior." *Neuroscience and Biobehavioral Reviews*, Vol. 4 (September 20, 1979), pp. 69-76.

Sargent, Shirley. *Galen Clark, Yosemite Guardian.* Yosemite, California: Flying Spur Press, 1981.

Smyth, D.G., National Institute for Medical Research, London, England. "B-Endorphin and related peptides in pituitary, brain, pancreas, and antrium." *British Medical Journal*, Vol. 39, No. 1 (1983), pp. 25-30.

Vaughan, Peter F.T., Glasgow University, Scotland. "The effect of neuropeptides on neurotransmitter biochemistry in the CNS." *Cellular and Molecular Biology*, Vol. 28, No. 4 (1982), pp. 369-382.

Bibliography

Wall, P.D., and C.J. Woolf, University College, London, England. "What we don't know about pain." Vol. 287 (September, 1980), pp. 185-186.

Chapter Five

Aronoff, G.M., R. Kamen, and W.O. Evans, Boston Pain Unit, Massachusetts Rehabilitation Hospital. "The relaxation response: a behavioral answer for chronic painpatients."*Behavioral Medicine* (1981), pp. 20-22.

Auden, W.H., and N.H. Pearson, eds. *Poets of the English Language, Vol. 5.* New York: The Viking Press, 1950.

Bellack, A.S., M. Hersen, and J. Himmelhoch, University of Pittsburgh, Pennsylvania. "Social skills training compared with pharmacotherapy and psychotherapy in the treatment of unipolar depression." *American Journal of Psychiatry*, Vol. 138, No. 12 (1981), pp. 1562-1567.

Buscaglia, Leo. *Living, Loving and Learning.* New York: Ballantine Books, 1982.

Carr, Daniel B., Harvard Medical School, Boston, Massachusetts. "Endrogenous opiods and fever: a hypothesis." *Perspectives in Biology and Medicine*, Vol. 23, No. 1 (Autumn, 1979), pp. 1-16.

Carter, James P., Tulane University, New Orleans, Louisiana. "Unhealthy habits: science seeks the cause." *Rx Being Well*, Vol. 2, No. 3 (May/June,1984), pp. 64-68.

Cassens, G., et al, Harvard University, Boston, Massachusetts. "Alterations in brain Norepinephrine metabolism induced by environmental stimuli previously paired with inescapable shock." *Science*, Vol. 209 (September, 1980), pp. 1138-1140.

Cousins, Norman. *Anatomy of An Illness, As Perceived by a Patient.* New York: W.W. Norton, 1979.

Field, Joanna. *A Life of One's Own.* Los Angeles: J.P. Tarcher, Inc., 1981.

Fraioli, F., et al, Universita di Roma, Rome, Italy.

"Physical exercise stimulates marked concomitant release of B-Endorphin and ACTH in peripheral blood in
man." *Experimentia,* Vol. 36 (1980), pp. 987-989.

Glaser, William. *Positive Addiction.* New York: Harper
and Row, 1976.

Goldstein, Avram, Stanford University, Palo Alto, California. "Thrills in response to music and other stimuli."
Physiological Psychology, Vol. 8, No. 1 (1980), pp. 126-
129.

Holmes, T.H. and M. Masuda. "Life change and illness susceptibility." Paper presented as part of *Symposium on
Separation and Depression: Clinical and Research Aspects.* Chicago, Illinois. December, 1970.

Howe, Herbert M. *Do Not Go Gentle.* New York: W.W.
Norton and Co., 1981.

Keller, Helen. *The Story of My Life.* New York: Macmil-
lan, 1964.

Knight, James A., Louisiana State University School of
Medicine. "Spiritual psychotherapy and self-
regulation." *Inner Balance, the Power of Holistic Healing,* ed. E.M. Goldwag. Englewood Cliffs, New Jersey:
Prentice-Hall, Inc., 1979.

Konner, Melvin. *The Tangled Wing, Biological Constraints
on the Human Spirit.* New York: Holt, Rinehart, and
Winston, 1982.

Lingerman, Hal A. *The Healing Energies of Music.* Whea-
ton, Illinois: Quest Books, 1983.

Marek, G., *Beethoven: a biography of a genius.* New York:
Funk and Wagnalls, 1969.

Mickley, G.A., et al, U.S. Air Force Academy, Colorado
Springs, Colorado. "Endrogenous opiates mediate radi-
ogenic behavioral change." *Science,* Vol. 220 (June 10,
1983), pp. 1185-1186.

Moody, Raymond. *Laugh After Laugh, the Healing Power
of Humor.* Jacksonville, Florida: Headwaters Press,
1978.

Neary, J. "A rocky try at reshaping lives." *People,* Vol. 19,

Bibliography

No. 32 (May 9, 1983), pp. 33-35.

Newhouse, Flower A. *The Journey Upward,* Athene Bengtson, ed. Escondido, California: The Christward Ministry, 1978.

"Nitrous oxide eases pain." United Press International, July 31, 1983.

Pelletier, Kenneth R. *Toward a Science of Consciousness.* New York: Dell Publishing Co., 1978.

Prigogine, Ilya. *From Being To Becoming.* San Fransisco: W.H. Freeman and Co., 1980.

Ryan, S.M., A.P. Arnold, and R.P. Elde, University of California, Los Angeles, and University of Minnesota, Minneapolis. "Enkephalin-like immunoreactivity in vocal control regions of the zebra finch brain." *Brain Research,* Vol. 229 (1981), pp. 236-240.

Stein, L. and J.D. Belluzzi, University of California, Irvine. "Brain Endorphins and the sense of well-being: a psychobiological hypothesis." *Advances in Biochemical Psychopharmacology, Vol. 18,* eds. E. Costa, and M. Trabucchi. New York: Raven Press, 1978, pp. 299-311.

Teale, Edwin W., ed. *The Wilderness World of John Muir.* Boston: Houghton Mifflin Co., 1954.

Wilber, Kenneth, ed. *The Holographic Paradigm, Exploring The Leading Edge of Science.* Boulder, Colorado: Shambala Publications, Inc., 1982.

Wingerson, Lois. "Training the Mind To Heal." *Discover,* Vol. 3, No. 5 (May, 1982), pp. 80-85.

❊ ❊ ❊

— Index —

Index

Crib death, 61-62,
Criminal behavior,
  rehabilitation, 168, 171-172,
  reinforced, 76,
Crohn's disease, 85,

Deep-breathing,
  as therapy, 107,
Demerol, 153,
Dendrites, 12-13, 26, 31-32,
  and change, 137,
  and enrichment, 129, 132,
  142, 177, 180, 185,
  and longevity, 119-120,
  150, 179,
  and stimulus, 124, 125,
  139, 144 -145, 188,
  growth of, 115-117, 196,
Denko, C., 86,
Dependence, 17, 47, 76, 88,
  125,
Depression,
  and change, 93,
  and Endorphins, 1, 56-61,
  125,
  and immunity, 97,
  therapy for, 37, 65-66,
Diamond, M., 113-116, 125,
  137,
Disbelief, 146,
  and pain, 128,
Disease, 9-10, 195,
  and distress, 70, 151,
  freedom from, 33, 123,
  potential, 35,
Distress, 157, 195,

and Endorphins, 125, 128,
  140, 168,
and exercise, 159,
and failure, 81,
and helplessness, 151,
and memory, 101, 180,
defined, 70, 77-78,
freedom from, 123, 174,
perceptions of, 120, 125, 144,
  171,
Dopamine, 50,
Dubos, R., 33,
Duggan, A.W., 126,

Endicott, J., 58,
Enkephalin, 8, 75, 85, 126,
  196,
Enrichment, 196,
  and belief, 129, 192-193,
  and change, 144, 149, 179
  and Endorphins, 140,
  and exercise, 158-162,
  and healing, 141, 177,
  and nature, 146, 171,
  experiment with, 113-116,
  135,
Epinephrine, 50,
Euphoria, 196,
  addiction to, 46,
  and alcohol, 49,
  and change, 164-168,
  and eating, 42,
  and Endorphins, 1-2, 7, 9,
  12, 15, 18-19, 22, 29, 111-125, 139, 147, 183,
  and exercise, 15-16,
  and exploration, 136, 142,

Index

Index

Index

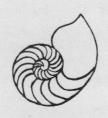

To order additional copies write —
Synthesis Press
P.O. Box 1141
San Marcos, CA, 92069

About the Authors

To bring you this inspiring book about Endorphins, Deva and James Beck have combined their multiple talents. Trained as both nurses and teachers, they are uniquely qualified to translate scientific discoveries into ideas that laypeople can use on a daily basis. The Becks have spent more than twenty years studying the fields of holistic health and body/mind research—documenting their relevance within traditional medical models—including health management, education, psychiatry, critical care, emergency medicine, rehabilitation, and hospice.

As public speakers, the Becks have widely shared wellness topics and Endorphin research in workshops and seminar formats, showing how Endorphin knowledge illuminates and unifies such popular concepts as stress management, self-help, alternative healing, and the body/mind connection. As lovers of life, the authors elevate the topic of Endorphins—into a creative celebration of the best life has to offer.